Application of Nursing Process

A Step-by-Step Guide

Application of Nursing Process

A Step-by-Step Guide

Rosalinda Alfaro, R.N., M.S.N.

Adjunct Instructor
Delaware County Community College
Department of Nursing
Media, Pennsylvania

Staff Nurse
Intensive Care Units
Paoli Memorial Hospital
Paoli, Pennsylvania

J. B. Lippincott Company   Philadelphia
London   Mexico City   New York   St. Louis   São Paulo   Sydney

Acquisitions Editor: Patricia L. Cleary
Developmental Editor: Joyce Mkitarian
Copy Editor: Mary Frawley
Indexer: Sandra King
Design Director: Tracy Baldwin
Designer: Anne O'Donnell
Production Editor: Rosanne Hallowell
Compositor: Circle Graphics
Text Printer/Binder: R. R. Donnolley & Sons Company, Inc.
Cover Printer: Philips Offset Company, Inc.

6 5 4 3

Library of Congress Cataloging-in-Publication Data

Alfaro, Rosalinda.
    Application of nursing process.

    Includes bibliographies and index.
    1. Nursing—Handbooks, manuals, etc.   I. Title.
[DNLM: 1. Nursing Process—methods. WY 100 A 385a]
ISBN 0-397-54638-6

For my parents, Margaret and Jimmy.

And for Dianne, Tuck, Michael, Jim, Matt, Janet, Dennis, Daniel, Chris, Anne Marie, Ledjie, Heidi, Craig, Eric, Ellie, Holly, and Becky.

Consultants

My gratitude goes to the consultants listed below. Their time, suggestions, and critiques were invaluable in pulling this project together.

Ledjie Ballard, R.N., M.S.N.,
  C.R.N.A.
Formerly, Director of Lankenau
  Hospital School of Nurse
  Anesthesia
Philadelphia, Pennsylvania
Presently, Staff Nurse Anesthetist
Group Health Cooperative
Seattle, Washington

Lynda Carpenito, R.N., M.S.N.
LJC Consultants
Mickleton, New Jersey

Nancy Flynn, R.N., B.S.N.
Nursing Services Education
Bryn Mawr Hospital
Bryn Mawr, Pennsylvania

Joan Jenks, R.N., M.S.N.
Assistant Professor
Junior Level Coordinator
Department of Nursing
Jefferson University
Philadelphia, Pennsylvania

Rebecca Resh, M.Ed.
Coordinator of Educational Services
Centre for Head Trauma
Devereux Foundation
Devon, Pennsylvania

Sister Mary Carol Taylor, R.N., M.S.N.
Assistant Professor
Level One Coordinator
Department of Nursing
Holy Family College
Philadelphia, Pennsylvania

Preface

Although nurses have been using the nursing process for the past 2 decades, a tremendous amount of growth has been evident in the past 5 to 10 years. During this short period of time, the nursing process has evolved from a four-step procedure (Assessment, Planning, Implementation, and Evaluation) to a five-step procedure (Assessment, Diagnosis, Planning, Implementation, Evaluation). Nurses are beginning to describe the nursing activities that must be accomplished in a sequential manner in order to provide comprehensive, cost-effective, high-quality nursing care.

The rapid growth in information about the nursing process has produced a deluge of literature offering various points of view on how the nursing process should be implemented in nursing practice. Most nursing texts today incorporate the use of the nursing process to a degree, but few fully address each of the steps of the nursing process in any great detail. Many practitioners, educators, and nursing students are in search of a reference that will clearly describe the "state of the art" of the nursing process as of 1986. This book has been written with the intention of helping students and nurses to learn exactly what the nursing process entails, and how it should be applied in nursing practice.

Keeping in mind that students and nurses are expected to accomplish a large amount of reading and learning in a short period of time, I have presented the information succinctly, yet completely, using simple language and concrete examples. Whenever possible, guides and steps for performing certain aspects of the nursing process have been described in an outline format that can be used for quick reference (*e.g.,* "Guide for Performing Patient Teaching," and "Steps for Modifying the Care Plan"). Key points have been listed throughout the book to clarify and summarize what has been discussed. Practice sessions are provided to allow practice for performing the activities necessary for that particular phase of the nursing process.

This book contains all of the latest information concerning the nursing process. This includes a chapter on identifying nursing diagnoses using the list accepted by the North American Nursing Diagnosis Association, and new information on the process of planning nursing care.

In this book, the pronoun "he" is used to refer to the recipient of nursing care, and the pronoun "she" is used to refer to the nurse. The words "patient," "client," "person," and "individual" are used interchangeably. Whenever possible, I have used a fictitious person's name in place of "the client" or "the patient" to help us to keep in mind that each client or patient is an individual who has unique needs, beliefs, values, perceptions, and motivations.

As a practicing nurse and educator, I have tried to view the nursing process from many angles. At different times during a given month I have had the opportunity to view the nursing process through the eyes of an educator ("How *do* you teach this information to beginners?"), through the eyes of a student ("*What* does all this nursing process stuff *mean*?), and through the eyes of a practitioner ("*How* am I going to find the time to *do* all this?"). It is my hope that you will find that this is a book that bridges the gap between theory and practice, and that it is helpful for practicing nurses, as well as for students and educators. The nursing process is crucial to the heart of nursing, and I am eager for the time when we all (practitioners, educators, and students) become adept in using it as a vehicle to promote the growth of nursing practice.

Rosalinda Alfaro R.N., M.S.N.

Acknowledgements

I want to thank Nat and Louise Rochester for getting me started on the computer. Also, the following people for their belief in me, and for their contribution to my personal and professional growth: John Payne; Charlie Lindsay; Patti Cleary; Mary Jo Boyer; Lynda Carpenito; Heidi Laird; Ledjie Ballard; Diane Verity; Debbie Sowers; Annette Sophocles; Becky Resh; the faculty of Villanova University School of Nursing; and the present and past staff nurses of Paoli Memorial Hospital.

Special Acknowledgement

Special acknowledgement is given to Lynda Carpenito, R.N., M.S.N. for her time and expertise. All of the references that are labeled "verbal communication with" are the result of her willingness to clarify ideas that she has presented nationally in workshops, but has not yet published as of January, 1986.

Contents

Application of Nursing Process
A Step-by-Step Guide

Introduction

This book is intended to help make the nursing process make sense to you. I have purposely made the reading as easy as possible and have used many real-life examples and situations to make learning this content both interesting and relevant. I have also incorporated real-life situations into practice sessions that are specifically designed to give you the opportunity to become actively involved in using the steps of the nursing process. It is my hope that you will use this book in whatever way you find most helpful; for example, if you need added clarification, write it on the pages. Mark it up and make it yours. Do the practice sessions when you feel you need clarification. Omit them if you feel that you already understand the content. Example answers to the practice sessions are all in the back of the book for your referral, but try to do the sessions on your own before checking the answers. These practice sessions are for *your* benefit, and you should use them in whatever way you find most helpful.

The ANA standards for nursing practice (listed below) provide the foundation for the nursing process as described in this book.

American Nurses' Association Standards for Practice*

I. The collection of data about the health status of the client/patient is systematic and continuous. The data are accessible, communicated, and recorded.

II. Nursing diagnoses are derived from health status data.

III. The plan of nursing care includes goals derived from the nursing diagnoses.

IV. The plan of nursing care includes priorities and the prescribed nursing approaches or measures to achieve the goals derived from the nursing diagnoses.

V. Nursing actions provide for client/patient participation in health promotion, maintenance, and restoration.

VI. Nursing actions assist the client/patient to maximize his health capabilities.

VII. The client's/patient's progress or lack of progress toward goal achievement is determined by the client/patient and the nurse.

VIII. The client's/patient's progress or lack of progress toward goal achievement directs reassessment, reordering of priorities, new goal setting, and revision of the plan of nursing care.

*Abstracted from Standards—Nursing Practice. Copyright © American Nurses' Association, 1973.

☑ Assessment
☑ Diagnosis
☑ Planning
☑ Implementation
☑ Evaluation

1 Nursing Process Overview

☐ *Glossary*

Short, broad definitions are given here for the terms followed by asterisks. These will be defined in greater depth in later sections of the book.

Assessment* The first step of the nursing process during which data are gathered for the purpose of identifying actual and/or potential health problems

Diagnosis* The second step of the nursing process during which assessment data are analyzed

Etiology The cause of, or factors that contribute to, a problem, nursing diagnosis, or disease

Evaluation* The fifth step of the nursing process during which it is determined whether the goals of nursing care are achieved; the factors that are contributing to the success or failure of the plan are identified; and nursing care is either terminated or modified

Implementation* The fourth step of the nursing process, which involves putting the plan of care into action

Nursing intervention An action performed by a nurse to prevent illness (or its complications) and to promote, maintain, or restore health

Nursing process* An organized, systematic method of giving individualized nursing care that focuses on the unique human response of a person or a group of people to an actual or potential alteration in health

Medical treatment plan The plan used by physicians to treat diseases

Planning* The third step of the nursing process during which goals are set and a plan of nursing care is developed

In the following chapters, you will be able to study each step of the nursing process in depth. But for now, let's take a broad look at what the nursing process means. What is it? How does it work? Why should we use it?

What Is the Nursing Process?

Basically, the nursing process is an organized, systematic method of giving individualized nursing care that focuses on the unique human response of a person or group of people to an actual or potential alteration in health. In other words, it is a set of deliberate activities that the nurse should perform in a specific sequence to ensure that persons who require health care receive the best possible nursing care.

A short overview of the five steps of the nursing process follows.

Nursing Process Overview

☐ *Assessment:* During the assessment phase, you will need to *gather information (data)* to identify actual or potential health problems.

☐ *Diagnosis:* Once you are sure that the information you have gathered is correct, you are ready to *analyze the data.* This means that you must study the data you have collected for the following purposes:

> To identify actual or potential problems/nursing diagnoses
>
> To identify the cause, or etiology, of the problem
>
> To identify usual life-styles and coping patterns
>
> To determine which problems can be treated independently by a nurse, and which problems require that the nurse seek direction or orders from another health-care professional, usually a physician

☐ *Planning:* Once you have identified, or diagnosed, the problems, you are now ready to sit down with your patient and *make a plan of action* that will reduce or eliminate the problems and promote health. This plan of action will include the following:

> *Setting priorities*—(*i.e.,* What problems are the most important, and therefore must be accomplished first?)
>
> *Establishing goals*—(*i.e.,* Exactly *what* must be accomplished and *by when?*)
>
> *Prescribing nursing interventions*—You must decide what nursing actions/patient activities will help to achieve the goals that you and the patient have set.
>
> *Documenting the nursing care plan*—Other nurses need to know the plan of care that you have prescribed and the goals you expect to achieve.

☐ *Implementation:* Now is the time to put the plan into action. Putting the plan into action involves the following activities:

> *Continuing to collect information about your patient* to determine whether new problems are occurring and how the patient is responding to your actions
>
> *Performing the nursing interventions and activities* that you prescribed during the planning phase
>
> *Recording (charting) and communicating your patient's health status and response to nursing interventions.* You won't be there 24 hours a day, and other nurses need to know how the patient is doing and how the plan is working.

☐ *Evaluation:* You and the patient must determine how well the plan has worked and whether you need to make any changes in the plan of care. You must answer the following questions:

Have you and the patient achieved the goals that you set during the planning phase? (If so, have any new problems developed that have not been addressed? Could you achieve more than you had originally hoped for? Should you set new goals? What made the plan work? Is there anything you could have done to make it easier?)

Have you only partially achieved the goals, or perhaps not at all? (If so, why didn't you achieve your goals? Were the goals realistic? Was the patient committed to the goals? Are these goals still important? Did you have enough time? Did other problems arise that impeded your progress? Were your prescribed interventions appropriate? Did you consistently perform the interventions as prescribed? What changes are you going to make?)

Display 1-1 summarizes the five steps of the nursing process.

Display 1-1. *Steps of the Nursing Process*

Assessment . . . . Gathering information (data)

Diagnosis . . . . Analyzing data to identify problems/nursing diagnoses

Planning . . . . Making a plan of action

Implementation . . . . . Putting the plan into action

Evaluation . . . . Determining if the plan has worked

To remember the steps of the nursing process, remember the first letter of each of the steps (ADPIE).

Relationships among the Steps of the Nursing Process

The steps of the nursing process are closely related. *Each step is dependent on the accuracy of the step before it.* For example, it would be difficult to make a correct diagnosis if the assessment data were incorrect.

The assessment phase and the diagnosis phase are closely related and slightly overlapping because many nurses begin early interpretation and analysis of their data to formulate possible diagnoses as they are actually gathering the information. For example, if an experienced nurse notes that her patient has an irregular pulse, swollen ankles, and difficulty in breathing, she will probably begin to think, "this patient may have a heart problem" as she continues to assess the patient's vital signs. The diagram below shows the relationship between the assessment phase and the diagnosis phase.

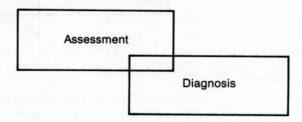

The diagnosis phase is closely related to the planning phase for two reasons:

1. The goals that are set and the interventions that are prescribed during the planning phase are derived directly from the problems that you have diagnosed. Therefore it is highly unlikely that your plan will be a good one if you have not correctly diagnosed the problems or have been vague in their description.

2. Nurses often begin the early stages of planning as they are identifying health problems. For example, a nurse may be analyzing the problem of powerlessness related to hospitalization, and at the same time, she may be considering possible interventions that might reduce the patient's feeling of powerlessness. The diagram below shows the relationship between the diagnosis phase and the planning phase.

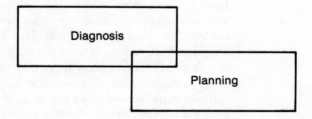

The planning and implementation phases are also closely interrelated because experienced nurses often begin to implement nursing actions before the planning phase is completed. For example, a nurse who observes that her patient is having trouble breathing may implement a plan by immediately raising the head of the patient's bed. This action is a result of a quick mental plan, and further planning may be necessary. The diagram below shows the relationship between the planning phase and the implementation phase.

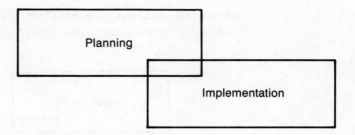

Ideally the fifth step of the nursing process involves determining whether you have achieved the goals set forth in the planning phase.

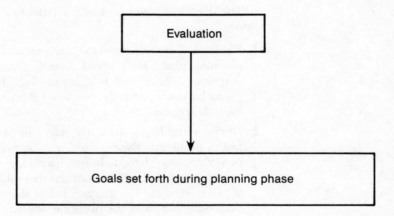

However, in practice, and especially if you are a beginning nurse, you should also be reassessing the client to be sure that there are no new diagnoses evident (*i.e.,* Did you miss any data during assessment? Did you miss a diagnosis?). If your goals were not achieved or were only partially achieved, you should be evaluating whether any new problems have arisen that would impede progress, whether your plan is a good one, and whether the plan was actually implemented. Having decided these things, you are ready for the final phase of evaluation—to terminate the nursing care if the problems are resolved and nursing is no longer necessary, or to change the plan of care to incorporate those changes that you and the patient have decided are necessary. Thus, you can see that evaluation actually involves three phases:

1. Evaluating goal achievement
2. Evaluating the other steps of the nursing process to determine what factors contributed to the success or failure of the plan of care
3. Terminating the nursing care if nursing is no longer needed, or changing the plan of care to incorporate necessary changes

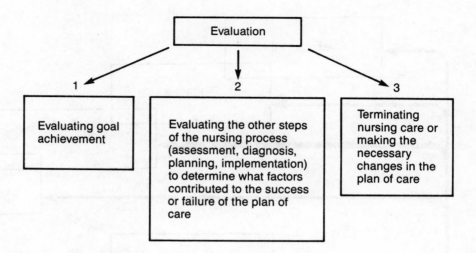

To summarize, the nursing process is a five-step cycle of activities that begins with assessment and culminates with evaluation. Note the example below.

☐ *Assessment:* You note that the person complains that his throat and mouth are dry. His temperature is elevated to 100° F. His record shows that he hasn't had anything to drink all morning. He states that he knows he should be drinking fluids, but he doesn't like water, especially when warm, and hates to keep bothering the nurses for juice.

☐ *Diagnosis:* You analyze the above data and decide that he probably has a *Fluid Volume Deficit related to insufficient fluid intake and fever.*

☐ *Planning:* You set a goal of drinking at least 2500 ml/day.

☐ *Implementation:* You offer preferred fluids at set intervals during a 24-hour period.

☐ *Evaluation:* You determine if he's meeting the established goal of drinking 2500 ml of liquid a day. If not, you decide why not, and make the necessary changes. If his condition is improved and he no longer has even a potential for *Fluid Volume Deficit* (*i.e.,* his temperature is normal), then you terminate the plan and allow the person to determine his own pattern of drinking fluids.

Study Figure 1-1 to clarify the relationships among all of the steps of the nursing process.

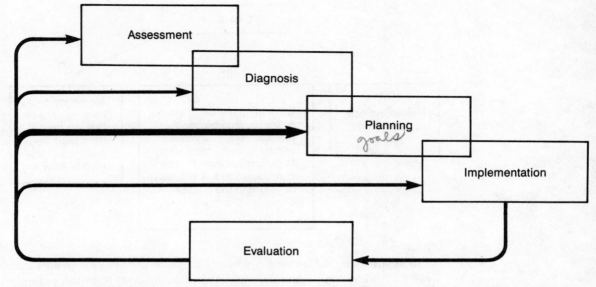

Figure 1-1. *Relationships among the steps of the nursing process. Each step of the nursing process is dependent on the accuracy of the step preceding it. The steps are also slightly overlapping. For example, you may begin the early stages of formulating diagnoses while you are actually performing the nursing assessment. You may be doing some mental planning as you are implementing the plan. The first phase of evaluation involves evaluating goal achievement, but you must also look at the entire plan to decide what factors are contributing to its success or failure.*

How Does the Nursing Process Work?

Using a problem-solving approach is the key to understanding the nursing process. Many of you will recognize the steps listed in Display 1-2 as a common method that you have been using for years to solve the problems that you have encountered in your own daily lives.

Display 1-2. *Steps of the Problem-Solving Method*

1. You encounter a problem of some sort and begin to collect information to see if you can understand the problem more clearly.
2. You study the information and identify just what the problem is.
3. You make a plan of action: "This is what I'm going to do about this problem."
4. You carry out the plan of action.
5. You evaluate whether the plan of action is helping to solve the problem. (You ask yourself, "Is this working? Is this problem really better? What else should I be doing to solve this problem?")

As you can see, the problem-solving method is very evident in the nursing process. Table 1-1 compares the steps of the nursing process and the problem-solving method.

Table 1-1. *Comparison of Nursing Process and Problem-Solving Method*

Nursing Process	Problem-Solving Method
Assessment—collecting data	Encountering a problem—collecting data
Diagnosis—analyzing data to identify health problems	Analyzing the data to identify exactly what the problem is
Planning	Making a plan of action
Implementation	Putting the plan into action
Evaluation	Evaluation of results

Why Should We Use the Nursing Process?

The nursing process provides a systematic and organized method of delivering nursing care. When all nurses consistently use the nursing process, the quality of nursing care is enhanced because it is less likely that there will be omissions and duplications in patient care. The nursing process encourages mutual goal setting and planning, with both the client and the nurse having input into the overall plan of care. This helps to make the client feel that he is an important part of a team that is working to accomplish common goals and encourages him to participate in decisions concerning his own health care.

Using the nursing process helps to create a nursing care plan that focuses on *human responses.* Unlike the medical treatment plan which focuses on *treating the disease,* the nursing process provides a treatment plan that nurses can use to *treat the whole person (i.e.,* this patient is a unique individual who is responding to his environment and health state in his own unique way, and who will require nursing interventions that are tailored specifically for him, not just for his disease). A comparison of the nursing process and a medical treatment plan is shown in Display 1-3.

Display 1-3. *Comparison of How a Nurse and a Physician May Gather Data About the Same Patient*

Physician's Data (Focuses on Disease)

"Mrs. Smith is experiencing an exacerbation in her rheumatoid arthritis that is causing increased pain and swelling in the joints of both hands."

Nurse's Data (Focuses on the Human Response to Health State)

"Mrs. Smith has pain and swelling in both hands, which has made it difficult for her to feed and dress herself. She states that she is fearful of losing her independence, cries easily, and repeatedly requests not to be placed in a nursing home." (The nurse focuses on the effects of the pain and swelling upon the patient's daily life, *i.e.*, the patient is having trouble feeding and dressing herself and is fearful of losing her independence).

Benefits of the Nursing Process

The use of the nursing process and nursing care plans helps to improve continuity of care. Each nurse has the benefit of reading a planned, organized nursing care plan before seeing the patient. This helps the nurse to "get a head start" in identifying health problems, and helps reduce frustration on the part of the patient because he is less likely to have to give repetitive information to each new nurse. The patient can then also be included in developing his own care plan and encouraged to participate in decisions about his own health care.

The nursing process provides for continual ongoing assessment and evaluation and therefore is not a static method of giving nursing care. The nursing process is dynamic and ever-changing as the patient's needs change or problems are resolved. Use of the nursing process promotes flexibility in giving total patient care.

Following an organized, systematic method of delivering nursing care helps the nurse to perform nursing activities in an efficient, goal-directed manner. This helps to reduce the frustration that can come from trying to give care in a haphazard, disorganized fashion. Nurses who implement the nursing process to direct their activities have the satisfaction of seeing results and making a difference in their clients' lives.

Display 1-4 summarizes the benefits of the nursing process.

Display 1-4. *Benefits of Using the Nursing Process*

1 Provides an organized method of giving nursing care

2 Prevents omissions and unnecessary repetitions

3 Provides for better communication

4 Focuses on the individual's unique human response

5 Promotes flexibility in giving individualized nursing care

6 Encourages participation on the part of the patient

7 Helps nurses gain satisfaction by getting results

□ *Key Points*   *Nursing Process Overview*

1. The steps of the nursing process can be remembered by using the mnemonic ADPIE (pronounced ăd'pī):

   Assessment

   Diagnosis

   Planning

   Implementation

   Evaluation

2. The nursing process utilizes a problem-solving approach that offers a systematic and organized method of delivering nursing care.

3. Each step of the nursing process is dependent on the accuracy of the step preceding it (*e.g.,* correct diagnosis is dependent on correct assessment data).

4. The medical treatment plan differs from the nursing treatment plan in the following ways:

   The nursing treatment plan focuses on treating the individual's unique human response to an actual or potential alteration in health.

   The medical treatment plan focuses on treating the disease.

□ *Practice Session*   *Nursing Process Overview*
                         (suggested answers on page 160)

1. Discuss the difference between the nursing process and the medical treatment plan.

(continued)

☐ *Practice Session*   2. List and define the steps of the nursing process.

3. List three advantages of using the nursing process.

☐ *Bibliography*   American Nurses' Association: Standards of Nursing Practice. Kansas City, MO, American Nurses' Association, 1973

American Nurses' Association: Nursing: A Social Policy Statement. Kansas City, MO, American Nurses' Association, 1980

Atkinson L, Murray M: Understanding the Nursing Process. New York, Macmillan, 1979

Carpenito L: Nursing Diagnosis: Application to Clinical Practice. Philadelphia, JB Lippincott, 1983

Gordon M: Nursing Diagnosis: Process and Application. New York, McGraw-Hill, 1982

Griffith J, Christensen P: Nursing Process: Application of Theories, Frameworks and Models. St Louis, CV Mosby, 1982

Kozier B, Erb G: Fundamentals of Nursing: Concepts and Process. Menlo Park, CA, Addison-Wesley, 1979

Potter P, Perry A: Fundamentals of Nursing Concepts: Concepts, Process, and Practice. St Louis, CV Mosby, 1985

☑ Collecting Data
☑ Validating Data
☑ Organizing Data
☑ Identifying Patterns

2 Assessment

Standard I: *The collection of data about the health status of the client/patient is systematic and continuous. The data are accessible, communicated, and recorded.**

*Abstracted from Standards—Nursing Practice. Copyright American Nurses' Association, 1973

□ *Glossary*

Cue   Something that is noted by using the five senses (taste, touch, smell, sight, and hearing). A cue can either be subjective data or objective data

Data base nursing assessment   Comprehensive nursing assessment that is usually completed upon initial contact with the patient to gather information about all aspects of the patient's health

Focus nursing assessment   Nursing assessment that focuses on gathering more information about a specific problem that has already been identified

Inference   How someone *perceives* or *interprets* a cue (*e.g.*, one person may perceive an individual's silence as acceptance, while another may interpret it as defiance, depending on judgment)

Nursing assessment   The gathering of information (data) about an individual, family, or community to identify actual and potential nursing diagnoses/problems

Objective data   Information that is concretely *observable* (*i.e.*, information that can be readily and surely seen with the eye [observation], felt with the hand [palpation/percussion], heard with the ear [auscultation], tasted, or smelled). Some examples are vital signs; numerical lab reports, such as a blood sugar of 115; diagnostic studies, such as electrocardiograms and x-rays; a limb that is swollen; definite colors such as red or blue

Subjective data   Information that the patient or client actually tells the nurse during the nursing assessment (usually charted as "Patient states. . . .")

Validation   The process of making sure the information or data you have collected is factual or true

Assessment is the first step of the nursing process. Because all nursing decisions and interventions are based on the information gathered during this phase, you should consider this step to be very important. During the assessment phase you should be gathering as much pertinent information about the patient as possible. This process of gathering information will include the following activities:

1. Data collection
2. Data validation
3. Data organization
4. Pattern identification

Display 2-1 further describes the components of the assessment phase.

Display 2-1. *Components of the Assessment Phase*

Data collection: Gathering information about the patient or client

Data validation: Making sure that you know which data are actually fact and which data are questionable

Data organization: Clustering the data into groups of information that would help you to identify patterns of health or disease

Pattern identification: Making an initial impression about patterns of information, and gathering additional data to fill in the gaps to describe more clearly what the data mean

Data Collection

Data collection begins with the patient/client's first encounter with the health-care system. (This could happen on an outpatient basis, but for our purposes we will assume it is a hospital admission.) At the time of admission, a complete nursing assessment is accomplished, and pertinent data are documented on the chart and on the nursing care plan. Data collection *continues throughout the patient's hospital stay* as changes occur and new information is presented.

Let's take a look at this process of data collection and consider the resources and methods that you should be using to gather information about the health state of a given individual.

What Resources Should Be Used to Gather Data?

To gather data for the assessment phase of the nursing process, you will need to use as many resources as possible. This includes using information gathered from the following resources:

☐ Information gathered directly from the patient or client (This should be your primary source.)

☐ Information gathered from the individual's family or significant other

☐ Information obtained from the chart (lab studies, x-rays, medical history, physicians' orders, progress notes, written consultations, nursing documentation)

☐ Verbal and written information from other health-care professionals/workers who are working with the patient/client (e.g., nurses, social workers, physicians, physical therapists)

Display 2-2 lists the resources for gathering data.

Display 2-2. *Resources for Gathering Data*

1 Patient/client

2 Family/significant others

3 Medical records (chart)

4 Other health-care workers

How Should Data Be Gathered?

Data should be gathered by observation, interview, and examination, with special consideration given to the person's developmental age (*i.e.,* your method of observing, interviewing, and examining should differ for infant, toddler, adolescent, adult, and elderly patients).

Data collection begins with the *nursing interview* and the *physical assessment* that is completed upon admission to the hospital. It is during this initial *comprehensive admission assessment,* called the *data base assessment,* that you will gain vital information about all aspects of your patient's health. This data base assessment is a basis for your ongoing nursing assessment.

Unlike the comprehensive data base assessment, ongoing data collection often focuses on gathering information about a specific problem. This type of assessment is called the *focus assessment* (Aspinall and Tanner, 1985). For example, you may have learned on the initial data base nursing assessment that the patient suffers from constipation. In the focus assessment, you should collect data that help you identify some factors that might be contributing to the constipation. Display 2-3 shows the differences between the data base nursing assessment and the focus nursing assessment.

Display 2-3. *Two Types of Nursing Assessment*

1 **Data Base Nursing Assessment**	*2* **Focus Nursing Assessment**
Comprehensive, gathers data about *all aspects* of the client's health	Focuses on gathering data about *a specific problem* that has already been identified
Usually done on initial contact with the client	May be done on initial contact, but often a part of ongoing daily assessment

The following figures show examples of three data base nursing assessment forms. Figure 2-1 is organized according to the needs of a specific hospital. Figure 2-2 is organized according to Orem's theory of self-care and Figure 2-3 is organized according to Gordon's functional health patterns.

Display 2-4 on page 26 is an example of a focus assessment that is performed for a specific problem (in this case the problem is constipation).

(*Text continues on page 26*)

Figure 2-1.   *Sample data base assessment form (WNL = within normal limits).*
(Courtesy of the Wilmington Medical Center, Wilmington, DE)

Adult Nursing History
Admission Data Base

Date_____   Arrival Time_____

Arrived via: Ambulatory   Wheelchair   Stretcher
Admitted: From_____To_____
Information obtained from: Patient   Family (specify)_____   Other (specify)_____
Occupation_____ Members of household (specify)_____

Deferred │ I. **Communications Status**
         │   Level of consciousness: Alert   Drowsy   Confused   Nonresponsive
         │   Oriented   Yes   No   Specify_____
         │   Cooperative   Yes   No   Specify_____
         │   Language spoken: English   Spanish   Other (specify)_____
         │   Speech: Clear   Slurred   Aphasic   Garbled   Unable to speak
         │   Ability to express self verbally: Yes   No
         │   Ability to communicate: Appropriate   Inappropriate
         │   Hearing: WNL   Impaired   Deaf   Corrected   Lip-reads
         │   Vision: WNL   Impaired   Blind   Corrected
         │   Vertigo: Yes   No   Specify_____
         │
         │ II. **History**
         │   Reason for admission (patient's statement) _____
         │   _____.
         │   What does patient expect from this hospitalization? _____
         │   _____.
         │   Previous hospital experience?   Yes   No
         │   Existing medical problems:
         │   Diabetes   Cardiac disease   Arthritis   CVA   Other _____
         │   Hypertension   Cancer   Respiratory   Renal   _____
         │   Allergies: None known
         │   Medications   Yes   No   Specify_____Reaction_____
         │   Food   Yes   No   Specify_____Reaction_____
         │   Other _____
         │   Prostheses, appliances, or other devices:
         │   False eye   Braces   Dentures   Eyeglasses
         │   Artificial limbs   Hearing aid   Contact lenses   Cane
         │   Pacemaker   Wig   Walker   Ostomy
         │   Other (specify) _____
         │   Medications (prescription, over-the-counter)?   Yes   No   If yes, list below
         │   Medicine   Dose   Reason   With patient   Last dose   Prescribing physician
         │   _____
         │   _____
         │   _____
         │   _____
         │   _____
         │   _____

(Continued)

Figure 2-1. *(Continued)*

Deferred | **III. Functional Status** ☐ Bedrest ☐ BRP ☐ Up ad lib ☐ Immobile
☐ Right-handed ☐ Left-handed ☐ Ambidextrous

Motor Function: Specify

R Arm__WNL__Amputated__Spastic__Flaccid__Paresis__Paralysis__Other_____

L Arm__WNL__Amputated__Spastic__Flaccid__Paresis__Paralysis__Other_____

R Leg__WNL__Amputated__Spastic__Flaccid__Paresis__Paralysis__Other_____

L Leg__WNL__Amputated__Spastic__Flaccid__Paresis__Paralysis__Other_____

Patient's ability to ambulate: ☐ Independent ☐ Assistance needed _____

Gait: ☐ Stable ☐ Unstable

Bathe: ☐ Independent ☐ Assistance needed_____

Dress: ☐ Independent ☐ Assistance needed_____

Toilet: ☐ Independent ☐ Assistance needed_____

Eat: ☐ Independent ☐ Assistance needed_____

Swallow liquids ☐ Yes ☐ No   Swallow solids ☐ Yes ☐ No

Chew ☐ Yes ☐ No

Does the patient have problems/difficulty in:

Sleeping ☐ Yes ☐ No Specify_____

Eating ☐ Yes ☐ No Specify_____

Urination ☐ Yes ☐ No Specify_____

Defecation ☐ Yes ☐ No Specify_____

IV. Physical Assessment

Vital signs: Temp_____BP_____Weight_____Height_____

Pulse_____Strong_____Weak_____Regular_____Irregular_____

Pedal pulse_____Deferred_____

Pupils: ☐ Equal ☐ Unequal

Left: ·· • • ● ● ● Reactive to light
Left ☐ Yes ☐ No Specify_____

Right: ·· • • ● ● ● Right ☐ Yes ☐ No Specify_____

Eyes: ☐ Clear ☐ Draining ☐ Reddened ☐ Other _____

Mouth: Gums ☐ WNL ☐ White plaques ☐ Lesions ☐ Other _____

Teeth ☐ WNL ☐ Loose ☐ Other_____

Skin:

Color ☐ WNL ☐ Pale ☐ Cyanotic ☐ Ashen ☐ Jaundice ☐ Other _____

Temperature ☐ Warm ☐ Cool   Turgor: ☐ WNL ☐ Poor

Edema ☐ No ☐ Yes Description/location _____

Lesions ☐ None ☐ Yes Description/location _____

Decubitus ☐ None ☐ Yes Description/location _____

Bruises ☐ None ☐ Yes Description/location _____

Reddened ☐ No ☐ Yes Description/location _____

Pruritus ☐ No ☐ Yes Description/location _____

Respiratory rate _____

Quality: ☐ WNL ☐ Shallow ☐ Rapid ☐ Labored ☐ Other _____

Auscultation: Specify

Upper right lobes ☐ WNL ☐ Decreased ☐ Absent ☐ Abnormal sounds _____

Upper left lobes ☐ WNL ☐ Decreased ☐ Absent ☐ Abnormal sounds _____

Lower right lobes ☐ WNL ☐ Decreased ☐ Absent ☐ Abnormal sounds _____

Lower left lobes ☐ WNL ☐ Decreased ☐ Absent ☐ Abnormal sounds _____

Is patient aware of diagnosis? ☐ Yes ☐ No ☐ Dx not established

What is the person most concerned about? _____

Summary Statement: _____

_____

_____

_____

☐ am

Date_____Time_____ ☐ pm _____RN

Figure 2-2.   *Data base assessment form organized according to Orem's theory of self-care. (With permission of Holy Family College Department of Nursing, Philadelphia, PA)*

Nursing History

I. Client profile
  A. Personal characteristics
    1. Name
    2. Age
    3. Sex
    4. Marital status
    5. Ethnic orientation
    6. Religious orientation
    7. Educational level
    8. Language
    9. Occupational history (type of job, duration)
    10. Interest, hobbies, recreational activities
  B. Current health orientation
    1. What do you consider to be healthy about you?
    2. What are your health goals?
  C. Family characteristics
    1. Family members/significant others (age, relationship to client)
    2. Type of family form
    3. Family structure
      a. Role structure
      b. Value systems
      c. Communication pattern
      d. Power structure
    4. Family function
      a. Affective function
      b. Socialization and social placement function
      c. Reproductive function
      d. Family coping function
      e. Economic function
      f. Provision of physical necessities
  D. Environmental characteristics
    1. Physical setting: home (characteristics, safety hazards, spatial adequacy, provision of privacy)
    2. Physical setting: neighborhood and community, including geographic mobility patterns; presence of environmental hazards
    3. Associations and transactions of the family with the community, and perception and feelings about neighborhood and community; include accessibility of health care facilities, human services
II. Universal self-care requisites
  A. Air
    1. Health habits
      a. Hygiene (bathing and grooming practices, oral hygiene, feminine hygiene, special cultural practices)
      b. Patterns of oxygenation (special aids)
    2. Review of systems
      a. Skin: rashes, pruritus, scaling, lesions, turgor, skin growths, tumors, masses, pigmentation changes or discoloration
      b. Hair: changes in amount, texture, character; alopecia; use of dyes
      c. Nails: changes in appearance, texture, capillary refill
      d. Breast: pain, skin changes, lesions, dimpling, lumps, nipple discharge, mastectomy

(Continued)

Figure 2-2.   *(Continued)*

    e. Respiratory system: nose (pain or trauma, olfaction, sensitivity, epistaxis, discharge); shortness of breath, dyspnea, chronic cough, sputum production, hemoptysis; history of asthma, wheezing, or noise with breathing

    f. Cardiovascular system: palpitations, heart murmur, varicose veins; history of heart disease; hypertension, chest pain, orthopnea

    g. Peripheral vascular system: coldness, numbness, discoloration, peripheral edema, intermittent claudication

B. Water
1. Health habits
    a. Patterns of fluid intake
    b. Fluid likes/dislikes
    c. Fluid temperature preferences
2. Review of systems
    a. Hydration: dehydration, excessive dryness, sweating; odors, edema, polydipsia
    b. Parenteral fluids (IV blood administration, hyperalimentation)

C. Food
1. Health habits
    a. 24-hour diet recall
    b. Food likes and dislikes
    c. Dietary modifications (cultural, religious, medical)
    d. Food preparation
    e. Meal environment
    f. Food budgeting
    g. Food supplements (vitamins, minerals, fluorinated water supply)
    h. weight gain/loss patterns
    i. Problems related to ingestion/digestion (special aids)
    j. Related prescribed or patent medicines
2. Review of systems
    a. Mouth: teeth, gums, tongue, buccae, chewing difficulty
    b. Throat: pain, lesions, dysarthria, dysphagia, history of strep infections
    c. Gastrointestinal system: pain, anorexia, nausea/vomiting, acid indigestion, ulcer history, polyphagia, present height–weight status

D. Elimination
1. Health habits
    a. Daily patterns (bladder, bowel)
    b. Aids (fluids, foods, medications, enemas)
2. Review of systems
    a. Bladder: polyuria, oliguria, dysuria, nocturia, incontinence, difficulty stopping or starting stream, force of stream, dribbling, pain or burning on urination, urinary tract infections
    b. Bowel: pain, diarrhea, constipation (acute or chronic), flatulence, hemorrhoids, stool characteristics (color, consistency, amount)
    c. Surgical opening: draining wounds, ostomies
    d. Genitalia: perineal rashes and irritations, lesions, unusual discharge (amount, color, consistency)

E. Activity and rest
1. Health habits
    a. Activity patterns: means of ambulation (safety concerns, aids); level of activity (home, work, leisure); regular exercise program
    b. Sleep/rest patterns: circadian rhythms; time and duration of sleep; use of supportive aids (sedatives, alcohol, pillows), devices (reading, music)

(Continued)

    2. Review of systems
      a. Musculoskeletal system: muscle strength/weakness, muscle tone, range of motion, pain, fatigue, swelling, stiffness, contractures
      b. Neurological system: numbness, tingling; discrimination between heat, cold, and touch; unusual movements (tremors, seizures); paralysis; dizziness, headache, loss of consciousness, memory changes; intolerance to heat and cold

F. Solitude and social interaction
    1. Health habits
      a. Communication
      b. Social interactions
      c. Sexuality: attitudes toward own sexuality (femininity/masculinity), sexual orientation, frequency of sexual activity, satisfaction with sexual activity, contraceptive measures
      d. Solitude: opportunities and selected activities during solititude
    2. Review of systems
      a. Ear: pain, discharge, tinnitus, decrease/increase in hearing, use of hearing aids
      b. Eye: pain, discharge, vision, corrective lenses, blurred vision, diplopia, night blindness, color vision
      c. Reproductive system:
        Male: number of offspring, infertility, venereal disease.
        Female: age of menarche, number of days in cycle, type and amount of flow, premenstrual tension, dysmenorrhea, hypermenorrhea/menorrhagia, polymenorrhagia, intermenstrual metrorrhagia, history of pregnancies, number of live births, number of abortions (less than 20 weeks gestation), number of still births, number of neonatal deaths, high-risk pregnancies, infertility, age of menopause

G. Hazards to human life, human functioning, and human well-being
    1. Personal safety practices
    2. Social habits (drugs, alcohol, tobacco, coffee–tea–coke; specify level of use)

H. Normalcy: promotion of human functioning and development within social groups in accord with human potential, known limitations, and the human desire to be normal
    1. Health habits
      a. health resources used (medical, dental, vision and hearing, screening programs, immunizations, counselling)
      b. Personal health practices (stress/anxiety management, meditation, relaxation techniques; self-breast exam, testicular exam)
    2. Self concept/image
      a. Body image (appearance, boundaries, limits, inner structure)
      b. Mental health:
        (1) attitude
        (2) affect/mood
        (3) thought processes (logical, coherent, perceptual)
        (4) sensorium and reasoning (levels of consciousness, orientation, memory, calculation, abstract thinking, judgment/insight, intelligence
        (5) locus of control
        (6) potential for danger (harm to self/others)
      c. Spirituality

III. Developmental self-care requisites
A. Life-cycle stage and related concerns (neonatal, infancy, toddler, pre-school, school age, adolescence, early adulthood, middle adulthood, childbearing, late adulthood)
B. Psychosexual stage (Freud)
C. Psychosocial stage (Erikson)
D. Intellectual stage (Piaget)
E. Moral stage (Kohlburg)
F. Conditions that promote or prevent normal development (life events, poor health, education)

(Continued)

Figure 2-2. *(Continued)*

IV. Health deviation self-care requisites
 A. Present deviation
 1. Perception of deviation
 a. Reason for contact
 b. Understanding of this current alteration in health status
 c. Feelings about present health status
 d. Specific concerns
 2. Coping mechanisms
 a. Past use of coping mechanisms to deal with similar alterations
 b. Current repertoire of coping mechanisms and their adequacy
 c. Concurrent stresses (life events)
 3. Effects of deviation on life style
 a. Psychological   c. Financial
 b. Physiological
 B. Past history of health deviations
 1. Adult illness
 2. Childhood illness
 3. Accidents/injuries
 4. Hospitalizations
 5. Allergies
 a. Drugs   c. Other
 b. Food
 6. Medications
 a. Prescription   b. Self-prescribed
 C. Family health history
 1. Relatives living or dead with similar health deviations
 2. Presence of any hereditary diseases (diabetes, hypertension, heart disease)

Display 2-4. *Focus Assessment*

(During the data base assessment the nurse has identified that the patient has complained about constipation.)

Problem: Constipation

Assessment:

Does the problem exist *now?* Are the signs and symptoms of constipation (*i.e.*, hard, dry stool; abdominal cramping; no recent bowel movement; difficulty passing the stool) still evident?

Are the symptoms better, worse, or the same?

What are some possible contributing factors? (Assess for adequate diet, activity, hydration, and previous use of laxatives, medications.)

(Text continues on page 32)

Figure 2-3. *Data base assessment form organized according to Gordon's functional health patterns. (With permission, Nursing Service Department, Bronson Methodist Hospital, Kalamazoo, MI)*

BRONSON METHODIST HOSPITAL
Kalamazoo, Michigan

Medical/Surgical–Critical Care
Admission Assessment

A. Name:_____

Prefers to be called:_____ Age:_____

Date:_____ Time of arrival to unit:_____

Mode of admission:_____

I.D. bracelet on and coincides with addressograph: ☐ Yes ☐ No Information given by:_____

If unable to reach next of kin/legal guardian, contact:_____ Phone:_____

Valuables (list and state disposition):_____

Admitted from: ☐ Home ☐ Nursing Home ☐ Assisted Living ☐ Foster Care ☐ Senior Citizens' Apartments ☐ Other

  Facility Name:_____ Adm. Medical Diagnosis:_____

(DEMOGRAPHIC DATA — left margin)

B. Ht _____ Wt:_____ Kg

Temp:_____ ☐ Oral ☐ Ax. ☐ Rectal

Pulse:_____ ☐ Reg. ☐ Irreg.

Resp.:_____ ☐ Reg. ☐ Irreg.

BP: Left:_____

  ☐ Lying ☐ Sitting ☐ Standing

Right:_____

  ☐ Lying ☐ Sitting ☐ Standing

(VITAL SIGNS — left margin)

C. (The following have been explained):

Call system/bed-bathroom	☐ Yes ☐ N/A	Floor restrictions	☐ Yes ☐ N/A
Bed operation/siderails	☐ Yes ☐ N/A	Visitation Policy	☐ Yes ☐ N/A
Bathroom/bedpan-urinal	☐ Yes ☐ N/A	Lounge	☐ Yes ☐ N/A
TV/CH2/telephone	☐ Yes ☐ N/A	Newspaper/mail	☐ Yes ☐ N/A
Meal/cafeteria hours	☐ Yes ☐ N/A	Siderails policy	☐ Yes ☐ N/A
Smoking policy	☐ Yes ☐ N/A	Chaplain services	☐ Yes ☐ N/A

  Signature:_____

(ORIENTATION TO UNIT — left margin)

D. **Health Patterns Assessment:** Complete information, **including patient's words.** Indicate N/A if non-applicable. Circle, code, or check all other findings as appropriate.

1. Reason for hospitalization/chief complaint:_____

_____

Recent illness/exposure to communicable disease:_____

_____

Previous hospitalizations/surgeries:_____

_____

What other health problems have you had?_____

_____

_____

Things done to manage health:_____

_____

Statement of patient's general appearance (include condition of hair, skin, nails):_____

_____

_____

Tobacco use: ☐ Yes ☐ No ☐ Used to smoke:_____

EtOH use:_____

Allergies: ☐ Yes (list with reaction experienced) ☐ No

Food:_____

Medications/anesthetics:_____

Other (e.g., wool, tape, pollens):_____

_____

(HEALTH PERCEPTION/HEALTH MANAGEMENT — left margin)

FORM 102 (Revised 10/84) — Page 1

(Continued)

Figure 2-3. *(Continued)*

Patient's Name: _____ Hospital No.: _____ Date: _____

Medications: (e.g., prescript., non-prescript.) ☐ Yes ☐ No Did you bring? ☐ Yes ☐ No Taken home? ☐ Yes ☐ No ☐ N/A

NAME	DOSE	SCHEDULE	REASON	PRESCRIBING PHYSICIAN

Have you been taking your medication(s) as prescribed? _____

OTHER PERTINENT DATA: _____

initials

2. Special diet? _____ Supplements: _____

Pattern of daily food/fluid intake: _____

Appetite: _____ Wt. loss/gain: _____

Nausea/Vomiting: _____

GI pain: _____

Condition of oral mucous membranes: _____

Dental condition: _____ Dentures: ☐ Upper ☐ Lower ☐ Partial ☐ N/A

Skin: ☐ Warm ☐ Dry ☐ Cool ☐ Moist ☐ Other: _____

Turgor: ☐ Supple ☐ Firm ☐ Fragile ☐ Dehydrated ☐ Other: _____

Color: ☐ Pink ☐ Pale ☐ Dusky ☐ Cyanotic ☐ Jaundiced ☐ Mottled ☐ Other: _____

Edema: _____

Wounds/drains/dressings: _____

Skin problems (description and location): _____

I.V.'s: _____ ☐ N/A

OTHER PERTINENT DATA: _____

NUTRITION/METABOLIC

initials

3. Abd. tenderness/guarding/distention: _____

Bowel sounds: _____ Stoma (type): _____

Any problems with hemorrhoids/involuntary stool? _____

Usual bowel pattern (frequency, character, consistency, etc.): _____

_____ Date of last BM: _____

If problem, describe: _____

Use of anything to manage bowels (e.g., laxatives, enemas, suppositories, "home remedies", anti-diarrheals): _____

Usual urinary pattern (frequency, character, amount, incontinence, nocturia, etc.): _____

_____ Last void (time): _____

If problem, describe: _____

Perspiration/nocturnal sweats: _____

OTHER PERTINENT DATA: _____

ELIMINATION

initials

(Continued)

4.

CARDIO-VASCULAR STATUS

Peripheral pulses: _____
_____ □ N/A

Neurovascular check (e.g., capillary refill): _____
_____
_____

Chest pain/radiation: _____
_____

Jugular vein distention: □ Yes □ No
Hx of murmur: □ Yes □ No
Pacemaker: □ Yes □ No
Presence of A-V Shunt: _____ □ No
Arterio-venous bruit: _____ □ N/A

Monitor/rhythm: _____ □ N/A
Hemodynamic monitoring: _____ □ N/A

ACTIVITY / EXERCISE

RESPIRATORY STATUS

Respiratory pattern: □ No problem □ Dyspnea □ Nocturnal Dyspnea □ S.O.B. at rest
□ S.O.B. on exertion: _____ □ Other: _____
Lung sounds: _____ Use of accessory muscles? □ Yes □ No
Cough/production: _____ O$_2$ supplement: _____ □ N/A
Resp. tubes (e.g., ET, trach, chest/describe secretions/drainage): _____ _____
_____ □ N/A
Ventilatory assistance: _____ □ N/A

ACTIVITIES OF DAILY LIVING/MOBILITY STATUS

Use the **Activity Level Code** below to assess admission statuses:

	ADL Status		**Mobility Status**	
0–total independence	Feeding_____	Meal Preparation_____	Bed mobility_____	
1–assist with device	Bathing_____	Cleaning_____	Cart transfer_____	
2–assist with person	Dressing_____	Shopping_____	Chair/toilet transfer_____	
3–assist with device & person	Grooming_____	Laundry_____	Ambulation_____	
4–total dependence	Toileting_____	Other_____	R.O.M._____	

Handedness: □ Right □ Left
Able to use? □ Yes □ No
Reasons for ADL/Mobility limitations: _____
_____ □ N/A
Devices used for assist: _____ □ N/A
Do you need assistance with transportation? □ Yes □ No If "Yes", specify: _____
Where do you plan to be discharged? _____ Will you need assistance? □ Yes □ No
If "Yes", describe: _____
OTHER PERTINENT DATA: _____
_____

	initials

5.

Level of consciousness: _____ Oriented to: □ Person □ Place □ Time
Behaviors (describe): _____
Hx of epilepsy/seizures/Parkinson's, etc.: _____

COGNITIVE / PERCEPTUAL

REFLEXES

Reflexes: □ No problem □ Problem (If "No problem", do not complete this section.)
Eyes: Pupil size: r_____ l_____ Equal? □ Yes □ No Reaction to light: r_____ l_____
Accommodation: r_____ l_____ Deviation: _____
Handgrasp: r_____ l_____ Gag: _____ Swallow: _____
Movement of extremities: _____

SENSORIUM

Eyes/sight:	□ No problem □ Deficit: _____ Aid: _____
Ears/hearing:	□ No problem □ Deficit: _____ Aid: _____
Nose/smell:	□ No problem □ Deficit: _____
Tongue/taste:	□ No problem □ Deficit: _____
Skin/touch:	□ No problem □ Deficit: _____
Numbness/tingling:	□ No problem □ Deficit: _____
Dizziness:	□ No problem □ Deficit: _____

FORM 102 (Revised 10/84) — Page 3

(Continued)

Figure 2-3 (Continued)

Patient's Name: _____ Hospital No.: _____ Date: _____

COGNITIVE/PERCEPTUAL

PAIN

Pain: ☐ No problem ☐ Problem (If "No problem", do not complete this section.)
If "Problem", describe location, type, intensity, onset, duration: _____
_____
_____

Methods of pain management: _____
_____

COGNITION

Primary language: _____ Speech deficit: _____ Aid: _____
Any learning difficulties? _____
OTHER PERTINENT DATA: _____
_____ | initials

6. Usual sleep/rest pattern: _____

SLEEP/REST

Adequate? ☐ Yes ☐ No Factors affecting sleep/rest: _____
Methods to promote sleep: _____
Hx of sleep disturbances: _____
OTHER PERTINENT DATA: _____ | initials

7. Are there any ways you feel differently about yourself since you've been ill/hospitalized? _____

SELF-PERCEPTION SELF-CONCEPT

_____
_____
Description of non-verbal behaviors: _____
OTHER PERTINENT DATA: _____ | initials

8. Marital status: _____ Children: _____

ROLE/RELATIONSHIP

Do you live? ☐ Alone ☐ With family ☐ Other: _____
Family feelings regarding hospitalization: _____
Who are the people that will help you most at this time? _____
Are you presently employed? ☐ Yes ☐ No Occupation: _____ ☐ N/A
Are you presently in school? ☐ Yes ☐ No Will illness/hospitalization interfere? _____ ☐ N/A
Upon discharge, if necessary, will you be able to afford?
       Medications: ☐ Yes ☐ No   Supplies: ☐ Yes ☐ No   Medical Care: ☐ Yes ☐ No
OTHER PERTINENT DATA: _____ | initials

9. Female: ☐ N/A   Menopausal: ☐ Yes ☐ No   Menstrual pattern: _____ ☐ N/A

SEXUALITY/REPRODUCTIVE

  Problems/changes: _____
Date of L.N.M.P. _____ ☐ N/A Possibly pregnant? ☐ Yes ☐ No ☐ N/A
Pregnancy history: _____
Use of birth control measure ☐ Yes ☐ No ☐ N/A Type: _____
  Any problems with use? _____
Monthly self-breast exam? ☐ Yes ☐ No ☐ N/A
Vaginal discharge/bleeding/lesions: _____
  Receiving medical attention? ☐ Yes ☐ No ☐ N/A
OTHER PERTINENT DATA: _____ | initials

Male: ☐ N/A   Prostate problems? _____
Monthly self-testicular exam? ☐ Yes ☐ No ☐ N/A
Penile discharge/bleeding/lesions: _____
  Receiving medical attention? ☐ Yes ☐ No ☐ N/A
OTHER PERTINENT DATA: _____ | initials

FORM 102 (Revised 10/84) — Page 4

(Continued)

10. Have you experienced any recent stressful situations in addition to your illness/hospitalization? ☐ Yes ☐ No
If "Yes", please describe briefly:_____
_____
_____
_____

Are there any ways we can be of assistance?_____
_____
How do you usually manage stresses?_____
_____

What do you do for relaxation?_____
_____

Support groups/counselling resources used: _____
Were they helpful?_____ ☐ N/A
OTHER PERTINENT DATA: _____
_____

| | initials |

COPING/STRESS

11. Will illness/hospitalization interfere with any of the following?
Spiritual or religious practices? ☐ Yes ☐ No
Cultural beliefs or practices? ☐ Yes ☐ No
Familial traditions? ☐ Yes ☐ No
If "Yes", to any of the above, please describe briefly:_____
_____
_____
_____

Would you like your clergy or hospital chaplain to be contacted? ☐ Yes ☐ No ☐ N/A
OTHER PERTINENT DATA: _____
_____

| | initials |

VALUE/BELIEF

E. Include: a. Possible nursing diagnostic concept labels to consider for care planning.
           b. Possible referral resources to consider for discharge planning needs.
           c. Other pertinent information
_____
_____
_____
_____
_____
_____
_____
_____
_____
_____
_____
_____

| | initials |

IMPRESSIONS

DATE	TIME	INITIALS	SIGNATURES	
_____	_____	_____	_____	(1st Adm. R.N.)
_____	_____	_____	_____	(2nd Adm. R.N.)
_____	_____	_____	_____	(3rd Adm. R.N.)
_____	_____	_____	_____	(4th Adm. R.N.)

FORM 102 (Revised 10/84) — Page 5 .

The Nursing Interview

The nursing interview is an essential part of data collection. What you see and what you hear during the nursing interview will yield important information for your nursing assessment. The amount of pertinent data collected will depend on your interviewing skills (*i.e.*, your ability to establish a rapport, and to observe, listen, and question).

Establishing a rapport and learning to observe, listen, and question comes with practice, but the following guidelines for promoting a successful interview can be helpful in developing these skills:

☐ *Guidelines*   *Promoting a Successful Interview*

How to Establish a Rapport

☐ *Ensure privacy*. Provide a quiet, private setting without interruptions or distractions.

☐ *Use the person's name*. Introduce yourself and show a genuine interest in the individual's well being.

☐ *Explain your purpose*. Explain that the purpose of asking so many questions is to provide better nursing care by knowing more about the person and his family.

☐ *Use good eye contact*. Give the person your full attention.

☐ *Don't hurry*. Rushing may cause the person to feel that you are not interested in hearing what he has to say.

How to Observe

☐ *Use your senses*. Do you see, hear, or smell anything abnormal?

☐ *Notice general appearance*. Does the person appear well groomed, healthy, well nourished?

☐ *Notice body language*. Does the person appear comfortable? Nervous? Withdrawn? Apprehensive? What do you see?

☐ *Notice interaction patterns*. Be cognizant of the person's response to your interviewing style (for example, sometimes cultural differences will create communication barriers).

How to Ask Questions

☐ *Ask about the person's main problem first*. Asking questions about the problem that made him seek health care helps him feel purpose and expedience in your questioning.

☐ *Use terminology that the person understands*. Ask the person to repeat what has been said if you think he doesn't understand (for example, "Can you explain to me how you understand what we've said this morning?").

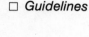☐ *Guidelines*

☐ *Use open-ended questions.* Ask questions that require more than a one-word answer. (See Display 2-5 for examples.)

☐ *Use reflection* (restating the person's own words in a question) to encourage him to expand on what has been said. (See Display 2-6 for examples.)

☐ *Don't start with personal or delicate questions.* Hold these questions until you get to know the person.

☐ *Defer questions that are not pertinent* if the person is too uncomfortable or upset. Only ask questions that are absolutely necessary.

☐ *Use an organized assessment tool to prevent omissions.* This is usually provided by the institution, or you can use any of the data base assessment tools shown in this book.

How to Listen

☐ *Be an active listener.* A nod or a glance of interest will help to encourage the patient to go on.

☐ *Allow the person to finish sentences.* Be calm and sympathetic, and don't rush him.

☐ *Be patient if the person has a memory block.* Give him time, and he may jog his memory when you ask related questions.

☐ *Give your full attention.* Discourage unnecessary interruptions.

☐ *For clarification, summarize and restate what has been said.* This reduces misunderstanding on the part of both the patient and the nurse.

Display 2-5. *Examples of Open-Ended Questions and Closed-Ended Questions*

Closed-Ended: "Are you happy about this?"
Open-Ended: "How does this make you feel?"

Closed-Ended: "Do you get along with your husband?"
Open-Ended: "How is your relationship with your husband?"

Closed-Ended: "Does this make you sick to your stomach?"
Open-Ended: "Describe the feeling that you are experiencing."

Display 2-6. *Examples of Reflective Statements*

Client states: "Sometimes I'm happy about how things are going, and sometimes I feel that everything is all wrong."

Reflective response: "So you feel happy some of the time, but sometimes things don't seem right?"

(*continued*)

Display 2-6 *(Continued)*

> *Client states:* "I wish I could be somewhere else?"
>
> *Reflective response:* " . . . Somewhere else?"

☐ *Key Points*   *The Nursing Interview*

1. The nursing interview is an important tool for gathering assessment data.
2. The patient himself should be considered the primary source of information. Additional important sources of information are the family, significant others, written records, and other health-care workers.
3. Promoting a successful interview involves establishing a rapport, asking probing questions, being a good listener, and being observant. (See *Guidelines: Promoting a Successful Interview.*)

☐ *Practice Session*   *The Nursing Interview*
(suggested answers on page 160)

1. Practice making open-ended questions. Rewrite each question below so that it is an open-ended question.

   a. "Are you feeling better?"

   b. "Did you like dinner?"

   c. "Are you happy here?"

   d. "Are you having pain?"

     e. "Are you and your wife happy?"

2. Practice clarifying ideas by using reflection and making open-ended questions. For each statement below, write a reflective statement and an open-ended question that would help you to clarify what has been said.

   a. "I've been sick off and on for a month."

   b. "Nothing ever goes right for me."

   c. "I seem to have a pain in my side that comes and goes."

   d. "I've had this 'funny feeling' for a week."

   e. "I feel weak all over whenever I exert myself."

The Nursing Physical Assessment

The nursing physical assessment should be performed in conjunction with the nursing interview. Physical assessment is accomplished by a thorough, systematic examination of the patient. This examination includes the following activities:

□ *Inspection:* Examination by careful and critical observation

□ *Auscultation:* Examination by listening with a stethoscope

□ *Palpation:* Examination by touching and feeling

□ *Percussion:* Examination by touching, tapping, and listening

The actual skills of physical assessment (how to inspect, auscultate, percuss, and palpate) come with practice, and it is important to maintain an active use of these skills in order to maintain competency. This type of practice is impossible to accomplish in a book like this, but it is possible to practice the mental steps of organizing a nursing physical assessment. For example, you may have questions such as, "Where do I begin? How do I know how to proceed with the exam? How do I know what's most important?"

The method of organization that you choose to perform the physical exam will depend on your own preference and the condition of the patient. For example, many nurses use a "head-to-toe" method for the initial examination. If you choose to use the "head-to-toe" approach, you begin by assessing the head and neck (eyes, ears, nose, mouth, and throat). Then you continue down the body to the thorax, abdomen, legs, and feet, in that order. Other nurses prefer to use a "systems approach" to gathering data. They begin by assessing the respiratory system (nose, mouth, throat, lungs) and continue by assessing the cardiac status, the circulatory status, neurological status, gastrointestinal status, genitourinary status, musculoskeletal status, and status of the skin (integumentary system). The order in which you examine the patient will depend on his state of health. For example, if you have a well client, you may choose to begin wherever you would like, so long as you always use the same method. (Always using the same method will help you to become methodical and lessens the likelihood of forgetting something.) On the other hand, if you have an ill patient, you should examine the area of the body where the problems are before you go onto the other parts of the body (*e.g.*, if the patient complains of abdominal discomfort, examine the abdomen first).

The following guidelines are suggested to help you when performing a physical assessment.

□ *Guidelines*   *Performing a Physical Assessment*

□ *Always promote communication* between yourself and the client. Introduce yourself, provide for privacy, establish a rapport, and use good interviewing techniques while you are performing the physical assessment (rather than working in silence).

□ *Don't rely on memory.* Jot down notes to be sure of accuracy.

□ *Choose a method of organizing your data collection* and always use it. Note the method suggested below:

□ *Guidelines*

1. *newo*
2. *- Resp*
3. *- CV*
4. *GI*
5. *GU.*
6. *MS- muscles & joints*
7. *- Skin.*

1. If there is an obvious problem or injury, *assess that problem first* (*e.g.*, if the person states, "I can't breathe," assess the respiratory system first).

2. Continue by assessing physical status in the following order*:

   a. Respiratory status: Breath sounds, rate, depth, cough

   b. Cardiac status: Apical rate, rhythm, heart sounds

   c. Circulatory status: Rate, rhythm, and quality of pulses (radial, brachial, carotid, femoral, dorsalis pedis)

   d. Status of the skin: Color, temperature, turgor, edema, lesions, hair distribution

   e. Neurological status: Mental status; orientation; pupillary reaction; vision and appearance of the eyes; ability to hear, taste, feel, and smell

   f. Musculoskeletal status: Muscle tone, strength, gait, stability, range of motion, gag reflex, bowel sounds, presence of distention, impaction, hemorrhoids (external)

   g. Gastrointestinal status: Condition of the lips, tongue, gums, teeth; presence of gag reflex; presence of bowel sounds; presence of abdominal distention or tenderness; impaction; hemorrhoids

   h. Genitourinary status: Presence of distended bladder, discharge (vaginal, uretheral)

□ *Key Points*

The Nursing Physical Assessment

1. The nursing physical assessment should be performed in an organized, systematic manner in conjunction with the nursing interview.

2. Physical assessment is accomplished by:

   Inspection: Examination by critical and careful observation

   Auscultation: Examination by listening with a stethoscope

   Palpation: Examination by touching and feeling

   Percussion: Examination by touching, tapping, and listening

3. The skills of physical assessment must be practiced frequently to ensure accuracy of data collection.

4. Physical assessment should be performed in an organized, systematic fashion. (See *Guidelines: Performing a Physical Assessment.*)

* Adapted from Carpenito's suggested data collection according to body systems (1983). This method of data collection actually prioritizes system assessment (*e.g.*, the respiratory status should be assessed before the cardiac status).

Organizing the Nursing Physical Assessment
(suggested answers on page 161)

Case History I

Mrs. Laird has been admitted with a medical diagnosis of gastro-enteritis. You enter her room for the first time today. She is lying on her side holding a cold rag over her head. Her eyes are closed, and you notice that she appears somewhat flushed. There is an emesis basin nearby that is empty. Her emergency room record states that she is 28 years old, married, and a homemaker.

1. List at least three things that you would want to assess first when performing the nursing assessment for Mrs. Laird.

2. Using an assessment tool of your preference, complete the data that are available in the history given above. If the data are not available, discuss how you may acquire the data. That is, what questions would you ask, and what systems would you examine?

Case History II

You have been told that Mr. Daniels had his gallbladder removed two days ago. You go into his room, and he is sitting in a chair near his bed reading the newspaper. There are two unopened packs of cigarettes on his night stand. He has a heparin lock for antibiotics in his left arm. When you ask how he is, he replies, "OK... except I'm so sore I can't move too much... then I start to cough and that kills me."

☐ *Practice Session*
1. List at least three things that you would want to assess first when performing the nursing assessment for Mr. Daniels.

2. Using an assessment tool of your preference, complete the data that are available in the history above. If the data are not available, discuss how you may acquire the data. That is, what questions would you ask, and what systems would you examine?

Case History III

In a clinical conference, or with another student or nurse, choose a real patient, and discuss how you would organize your nursing assessment for that particular patient. That is, what would you assess first, and how would you proceed?

Identifying Subjective and Objective Data

Data can be separated into two categories: subjective information and objective information. *Subjective information* is that information actually stated by the patient (*e.g.*, "I have pain."). *Objective information* is concrete, observable information that can be noted by any skilled nurse or physician.

☐ *Subjective data:* What the patient/client actually states. These are his *feelings and perceptions.*

☐ *Objective data:* Concrete, *observable* information such as vital signs, laboratory studies, and changes in physical appearance or behavior.

It is often difficult to remember the difference between these two categories. But, there is a trick! Remember the following:

☐ S–S   Subjective data are Stated.
☐ O–O   Objective data are Observable.

Note the examples of subjective and objective data listed in Display 2-7.

Display 2-7.

Subjective Data

"I feel sick to my stomach."

"I have a stabbing pain in my side."

"I wish I were home."

"I feel like nobody likes me."

Objective Data

Blood pressure of 110/70

Large mole the size of a quarter on side of face

Overtly obese

Walks with a limp

Ate all of his breakfast

Urinated 150 ml clear urine

☐ *Practice Session*   *Subjective and Objective Data*
(suggested answers on page 162)

Read the following case histories and answer the subsequent questions.

Case History I

Mr. Michaels is 51 years old. He was admitted two days ago with chest pain. His physician has ordered the following studies: electrocardiogram, chest x-ray, and complete blood studies including a blood sugar. These studies were just posted on the chart. When you talk with him, he states, "I feel much better today—no more pain. It is a relief to get rid of that discomfort." You think he appears a little tired or weary—he seems to be talking slowly and sighs more often than you would think is necessary. When his wife comes to see him, she is cheerful with him, but confides in you that he seems depressed or something. His vital signs are:

T: 98.6   P: 74 (regular)   R: 22   B/P: 140/90

□ *Practice Session*

1. List the subjective data noted in the case history given above (*i.e.*, what were you told directly?).

2. List the objective data noted in the case history given above (*i.e.*, what is Mr. Michaels' general behavior, and what information can be readily observed?).

Case History II

Mrs. Rochester is a 33-year-old mother of two young children. She is admitted with the medical diagnosis of diabetes. Today you enter her room, and she states, "The doctor says I have diabetes. I can't see how I could have diabetes. No one in my family has diabetes. I feel fine. . . . I don't see how I can make myself change the way I eat. Dieting drives me crazy. . . . That's why I weighed 190 pounds when you weighed me." On further questioning, she admits that she has been feeling unusually tired lately, and that she does seem to have to urinate more than usual. You check her chart and note that her fasting blood sugar was elevated at 144. Her vital signs are:

T: 98.1   P: 88 (regular)   R: 24   B/P: 144/88

1. List the subjective data noted in the case history given above (*i.e.*, what were you told directly?).

(*continued*)

☐ *Practice Session*   2. List the objective data noted in the case history given above (*i.e.*, what is Mrs. Rochester's general behavior, and what information can be readily observed?).

Case History III

In a clinical conference, or with another student or nurse, choose data from a real patient, and discuss and determine what are subjective data and what are objective data.

Identifying Cues and Inferences

When you are collecting data, you will be noting certain cues given by the patient and making inferences about these cues. A cue is data that are noted by using the five senses—taste, touch, smell, sight, and hearing (Carnevalli, 1983). When you are examining and interviewing a patient or client, you should note many cues that will contribute to your data collection. Some examples of cues are the examples of subjective and objective data in Display 2-7—the only way you could have noted that data is by using your sense of hearing or sight.

From each cue, you will make an inference; that is, you will perceive or interpret the cue in your own way. In other words, an inference is how someone perceives or interprets a given piece of data. What you infer from a given cue will depend on your own perception or judgment. Your nursing knowledge, your observational skills, and your own set of values and beliefs will influence how you interpret a given cue. For example, one nurse may infer that a client who is silent during a patient teaching session is listening attentively, while another nurse may infer that the person is not interested because he has no questions.

To clarify your understanding of cues and inferences, study the examples of cues with corresponding inferences shown in Display 2-8.

Display 2-8. *Cues with Corresponding Inferences*

Cue: Judy states, "I have trouble moving my bowels."
Inference: Judy is constipated.

Display 2-8 *(Continued)*

> *Cue:* Jeffrey is silent and withdrawn and has a sad face.
> *Inference:* Jeffrey is depressed.
> *Cue:* Mrs. Rayburn's blood pressure is 70/50.
> *Inference:* Mrs. Rayburn is in shock.
> *Cue:* Susan states, "I can't stand this pain any more!"
> *Inference:* Susan is experiencing unbearable pain.

□ *Practice Session*   *Identifying Cues and Inferences*
(suggested answers on page 162)

1. List the cues that you can identify in Case History I (Mr. Michaels, page 40).

2. List the inferences that you might make about the cues that have been identified.

3. List the cues that you can indentify in Case History II (Mrs. Rochester, page 41).

4. List the inferences that you might make about the cues that you have identified.

5. In a clinical conference (or with another student or nurse), choose data from a real patient, identify cues, and discuss the inferences you might make from the cues.

Validating Assessment Data

Validating data means making sure that the information you have gathered is factual or true. For example, you must make sure that the person means what he says—he may state he feels fine but may not really mean it. You must be sure that the inferences that you have made are correct. For example, the patient may offer the cue of "I'm having trouble moving my bowels." This may infer that he is constipated. However, further data should be gathered for clarification—the patient may not be constipated at all, but rather may be having painful bowel movements due to hemorrhoids.

So, you ask yourself, *"How can I tell what information is valid?"* The guidelines listed below are helpful in learning how to validate information that you have gathered.

☐ *Guidelines*

Validating Assessment Data

☐ Data that can be measured with an accurate scale of measurement can be accepted as factual (*e.g.*, a person who is measured to be 5 feet 6 inches and 145 pounds . . . a person who was born in 1935 . . . most laboratory studies).*

☐ Data that someone else observes to be so because of verbal and nonverbal cues may or may not be true. The nurse should attempt to verify this information by directly observing and interviewing the client.

☐ Validating data can be accomplished by the following ways:

1. *Recheck your own data* (*e.g.*, taking a blood pressure in the opposite arm or 10 minutes later).

2. *Check to be sure that there is no temporary factor that would alter the accuracy of your data* (*e.g.*, a person who has had a cup of hot tea or smoked a cigarette just before you took his temperature).

3. *Always recheck data that are extremely abnormal* (*e.g.*, use two scales to check an infant who appears much heavier or lighter than the scale states).

4. *Ask someone else*, preferably an expert, to collect the same data (*e.g.*, asking a more experienced nurse to check your patient's blood pressure when you are not sure).

---

* There is always the possibility of laboratory error or other factors that may alter the accuracy of the laboratory studies (*e.g.*, a fasting blood sugar that is done even though the person has eaten 1 hour before). Rechecking gross abnormalities should validate the studies.

□ *Key Points*   *Validating Assessment Data*

1. *Validating data* deals with making sure that the information you have gathered is factual or true (*e.g.*, making sure a person means what he says—he may state he feels fine, but may not really mean it). See Guidelines: Validating Data.

2. When performing a nursing assessment, nurses must first identify cues given by the patient. A *cue* is something that can be noticed by using the five senses (taste, smell, touch, hearing, and sight).

3. After identifying cues, the nurse makes certain *inferences* about what the cues mean (*i.e.*, the nurse identifies the cue and then infers [interprets] what it means).

Cue	Corresponding Inference
Hard stool	Constipation
T: 101.8F	Fever

4. *Correct inferences* about a given cue are dependent on the skill and knowledge of the nurse.

5. Objective data that someone else observes to be so because of verbal and nonverbal cues may or may not be true. The nurse should attempt to verify this information by directly observing, examining, and interviewing the client.

□ *Practice Session*   *Validating Assessment Data*
(*suggested answers on page 163*)

1. From the cues and inferences that you identified in Case History I (Mr. Michaels, page 40), indicate in three separate columns those that you feel are *certainly valid*, *probably valid*, and only *possibly valid*.

(*continued*)

2. For the data you list in the *possibly valid* and *probably valid* columns, identify some methods of clarifying if they are indeed true (*e.g.*, what other questions might you ask?).

3. From the cues and inferences that you identified in Case History II (Mrs. Rochester), indicate in three separate columns those that you feel are *certainly valid*, *probably valid*, and only *possibly valid*.

4. For the data you list in the *possibly valid* and *probably valid* columns, identify some methods of clarifying if they are indeed true (*e.g.*, what other questions might you ask?).

5. In a clinical conference, or with another student or nurse, choose data from a real patient, identify cues, and discuss the inferences you might make from the cues. Now discuss which cues and inferences are probably valid and what methods you might use for validation.

Organizing (Clustering) Assessment Data

After you have gathered and validated your assessment data, you will be ready to organize, or cluster, the data into categories of information that will help to identify actual and potential health problems, using a nursing focus. How you organize the data you have collected will again depend on your own knowledge, skill, and preference. Often, experienced nurses will organize the data mentally, while newer nurses find it helpful to organize the data on a separate piece of paper. As with the assessment tool for the gathering of data, many institutions and schools of nursing have a recommended or required method of organizing the data. Maslow (see Display 2-9) and Gordon (see Display 2-10) offer excellent methods of organizing data to maintain a *nursing* focus when clustering data that has been collected during the assessment phase of the nursing process. However, there are other good methods for organizing data collection, and you should use whatever method works best for you.

hierchy
of
needs

Display 2-9. *Organization of Assessment Data According to* Maslow

1. Cluster together data that pertain to physiological needs (survival needs).

    Examples: Food, fluids, oxygen, elimination, warmth, physical comfort

2. Cluster together data that pertain to safety and security needs.

    Examples: Those things necessary for physical safety (such as side rails on a bed) and psychological security (such as a child's favorite blanket).

3. Cluster together data that pertain to love and belonging needs.

    Example: Family members, significant others

4. Cluster together data that pertain to self-esteem needs.

    Example: Those things that make the individual feel good about himself (such as good grooming)

5. Cluster together data that pertain to self-actualization needs.

    Example: The need to grow and change and accomplish goals

Display 2-10. *Organization of Assessment Data According to Gordon (Functional Health Patterns)*

1. *Health-perception–health-management pattern.* Describes client's perceived pattern of health and well-being and how health is managed

2. *Nutritional-metabolic pattern.* Describes pattern of food and fluid consumption relative to metabolic need and pattern indicators of local nutrient supply

3. *Elimination pattern.* Describes patterns of excretory function (bowel, bladder, and skin)

4. *Activity-exercise pattern.* Describes pattern of exercise, activity, leisure, and recreation

5. *Cognitive-perceptual pattern.* Describes sensory-perceptual and cognitive pattern

6. *Sleep-rest pattern.* Describes patterns of sleep, rest, and relaxation

7. *Self-perception–self-concept pattern.* Describes self-concept pattern and perceptions of self (*e.g.,* body comfort, body image, feeling state)

8. *Role-relationship pattern.* Describes pattern of role-engagements and relationships

9. *Sexuality-reproductive pattern.* Describes client's patterns of satisfaction and dissatisfaction with sexuality pattern; describes reproductive patterns

10. *Coping-stress-tolerance pattern.* Describes general coping pattern and effectiveness of the pattern in terms of stress tolerance

11. *Value-belief pattern.* Describes patterns of values, beliefs (including spiritual), or goals that guide choices or decisions

(From: Gordon M: Nursing Diagnosis: Process and Application. New York, McGraw-Hill, 1982)

To show how data can be clustered according to different methods, the following two tables show clustering of the *same data* according to Maslow (Table 2-1) and according to Gordon (Table 2-2).

Table 2-1. *Data Organization According to Maslow*

Data

1. 21-year-old male
2. Married, no children *Se*
3. Occupation: Firefighter *Se Sa*
4. Ht: 6'1"; Wt: 170 lb
5. T: 98; P: 60; R: 16
6. B/P: 110/60
7. Unconscious from head injury
8. Spontaneous respirations
9. Lungs clear
10. History of seizures
11. Foley draining clear urine
12. Wife states he's always constipated
13. Tube feeding via nasogastric tube every 4 hours
14. Extremities rigid
15. Has reddened areas on both elbows
16. Allergic to penicillin
17. Wife states she feels as though she is falling apart
18. Wife states that before the ac- *Se* cident, he took pride in being physically fit
19. Wife states that they were considering converting to Catholicism before the accident

Data Organization by Maslow's Needs

Physical: 1, 4, 5, 6, 7, 8, 9, 10, 11, 12, 13, 14, 15, 16, 18

Safety/Security: 7, 10, 13, 17, 19

Love and belonging: 2, 17, 19

Self-esteem: 2, 3, 18

Self-actualization: 3

Table 2-2.   *Data Organization According to Gordon*

Data	Data Organization by Gordon's Functional Health Patterns
1. 21-year-old male	Health-perception–health-management pattern: 10, 18
2. Married, no children	
3. Occupation: Firefighter	Nutritional-metabolic pattern: 4, 5, 6, 8, 9, 11, 13, 15, 16
4. Ht: 6'1"; Wt: 170 lb	
5. T: 98; P: 60; R: 16	
6. B/P: 110/60	Elimination pattern: 11, 12, 13, 15
7. Unconscious from head injury	
8. Spontaneous respirations	
9. Lungs clear	Activity-exercise pattern: 14
10. History of seizures	
11. Foley draining clear urine	Cognitive-perceptual pattern: 7
12. Wife states he's always constipated	
13. Tube feeding via nasogastric tube every 4 hours	Sleep-rest pattern: 7
14. Extremities rigid	Self-perception–self-concept pattern: 18
15. Has reddened areas on both elbows	
16. Allergic to penicillin	Role-relationship pattern: 1, 2, 3,
17. Wife states she feels as though she is falling apart	Sexuality-reproductive pattern: 2
18. Wife states that before the accident, he took pride in keeping physically fit	Coping-stress-tolerance pattern: 17
19. Wife states that they were considering converting to Catholicism before the accident	Value-belief pattern: 19

☐ *Practice Session*   *Organizing Assessment Data*
(*suggested answers on page 163*)

1. Using a separate sheet of paper, choose a method of organizing your data collection and organize the following sets of data from the two case histories listed below.

☐ *Practice Session*

Case History I

1. Age 20
2. Single; lives with parents and two younger sisters
3. Occupation: College student
4. Religion: Protestant
5. Medical diagnosis: mononucleosis
6. T: 101; P: 110; R: 30; B/P 110/84
7. States he has a constant headache
8. States he is depressed because he is missing school and is worried that his girlfriend may "catch mono too"
9. Appetite poor
10. He is weak when he stands or walks.
11. Before illness he was in good health and ran 5 miles a day.
12. Urine output in the past 16 hours is 250 ml.
13. Last bowel movement was 5 days ago—states he "can't stand using the portable commode."
14. States he has a constant sore throat

Case History II

1. Age 36
2. Married, has three small children
3. Occupation: Landscape architect and homemaker
4. Religion: Episcopalian
5. Medical diagnosis: Pneumonia
6. T: 100; P: 100; R: 28; B/P 104/68
7. States she is concerned about how her husband is caring for the children—that it is "tough on him"
8. States she feels weak and tired all the time, but can't seem to rest because she keeps coughing all the time
9. Appetite poor. Is forcing fluids well (1000 ml per shift)
10. Before illness, she smoked a pack of cigarettes a day but has not smoked since hospitalization.
11. States she has always been in good health and has never had to be hospitalized (even gave birth at home)
12. States all the tests that have to be done make her nervous—she is worried about getting *AIDS* from needle sticks
13. Lungs have bilateral rhonchi. She coughs up thick yellow mucus.
14. Chest x-ray shows improvement over the past 2 days.
15. White blood cell count is elevated at 16,000.

Identifying Patterns and Filling in the Gaps

Once you have clustered your data into groups of information, you may begin to have some initial impressions about the presence of certain problems. For example, using Maslow's human needs as a method of organization, you may have clustered the following data under safety and security needs:

☐ 72-year-old male

☐ Is blind

☐ States that he's always hurting himself

☐ States that he uses a cane to detect objects in front of him

☐ Has visible bumps and bruises over arms and on head

The above data may suggest to you that this individual has a potential for injury. However, there is not enough data to determine *why* he has a potential for injury. Is it only because he is blind? Perhaps he is falling down because of weakness or dizziness. After all, if he's using the cane correctly, do you think he would be bumping himself all the time? These questions and thoughts that come to mind while you are gathering and clustering data should guide you to gather additional data to describe the problems more clearly. For example, with the above patient, you would need to use probing questions and ask the person to clarify *how* and *why* he keeps hurting himself. You may find that he actually is hurting himself because he is fainting or passing out for some reason. Perhaps he doesn't use the cane properly. Or perhaps he is a victim of abuse. All of these questions can only be answered by filling in the gaps in the information that you originally gathered. In other words, part of identifying patterns involves making an initial impression, noting gaps in the data you have gathered, and probing to fill in those gaps.

Your ability to identify the significance of certain data and make initial impressions will grow as your nursing knowledge grows. Taking this extra time to fill in any possible gaps in your data collection should help to ensure that you have gathered *all the pertinent data*. It will also help to prevent you from focusing too early during assessment and missing pertinent data. Once you have completed this final phase of assessment, you will be ready to go on to the next step of the nursing process: diagnosis.

☐ Key Points | *Organizing Data, Identifying Patterns, and Filling in the Gaps*

1. Choose a method of clustering groups of information that works for you, and use it consistently.

2. Once you have made an initial impression, take the extra time to ask yourself if there are any other factors that commonly contribute to this type of problem, and seek to learn if any of those factors are evident.

☐ *Key Points*

3. Use probing, clarifying questions to gather the data to fill in the gaps. For example, note the following questions:

"It seems to me that. . . .Is there any other reason this could be happening?"

"You told me that. . . . Could you be a little more specific?"

"When you say that . . . , can you describe to me exactly what happens?"

☐ *Bibliography*

American Nurses' Association: Standards of Nursing Practice. Kansas City, MO, American Nurses' Association, 1973

Aspinall M, Tanner C: Decision-Making for Patient Care, Applying the Nursing Process. New York, Appleton-Century-Crofts, 1985

Atkinson L, Murray M: Understanding the Nursing Process. New York, Macmillan, 1979

Bates B: A Guide to Physical Examination, 3rd ed. Philadelphia, JB Lippincott, 1983

Carnevalli B: Nursing Care Planning: Diagnosis and Management. Philadelphia, JB Lippincott, 1983

Carpenito L: Nursing Diagnosis: Application to Clinical Practice. Philadelphia, JB Lippincott, 1983

Gordon M: Nursing Diagnosis: Process and Application. New York, McGraw-Hill, 1982

Griffith J, Christensen P: Nursing Process: Application of Theories, Frameworks and Models. St Louis, CV Mosby, 1982

Kozier B, Erb G: Fundamentals of Nursing: Concepts and Process. Menlo Park, CA, Addison-Wesley, 1979

Maslow A: Motivation in Personality. New York, Harper & Row, 1970

Orem, D: Nursing: Concepts of Practice, 2nd ed. New York, McGraw-Hill, 1980

Potter P, Perry A: Fundamentals of Nursing Concepts: Concepts, Process, and Practice. St Louis, CV Mosby, 1985

☑ Analyzing Data
☑ Identifying Nursing Diagnoses
☑ Identifying Collaborative Problems

3
Diagnosis

Standard II: *Nursing diagnoses are derived from health status data.* *

* Abstracted from Standards—Nursing Practice. Copyright American Nurses'
Association, 1973

☐ *Glossary*

Category label   A title that gives a concise description of an individual nursing diagnosis (See Display 3-1)

Collaborative problem   An actual or potential problem that may occur from complications of disease, diagnostic studies, or medical or surgical treatment, and that can be prevented, resolved, or reduced through collaborative nursing interventions*

Defining characteristics   A cluster of signs and symptoms often seen with a certain nursing diagnosis

Diagnostic statement   A phrase that clearly describes a health problem.

Etiology   The cause or contributing factors of a health problem

Independent nursing intervention   A nursing action that is encompassed by licensure and law and that requires no supervision or direction from others (Potter and Perry, 1985)

Interdependent nursing intervention   A nursing action that requires direction or consultation from another health-care professional (often a physician)

NANDA   Acronym for the North American Nursing Diagnosis Association

Nursing diagnosis   An actual or potential health problem (of an individual, family, or group) that nurses can legally treat independently, initiating the nursing interventions necessary to prevent, resolve, or reduce the problem

Potential nursing diagnosis   A nursing diagnosis for which an individual is at high risk as evidenced by the presence of high-risk factors noted during the nursing assessment*

Possible nursing diagnosis   A nursing diagnosis that may or may not be present as evidenced by some ambiguous cues in the assessment data.* The ambiguous cues direct the nurse to gather more data to clarify what the cues mean and to confirm whether the defining characteristics for that diagnostic category are indeed present.

Once you have completed a full nursing assessment of your patient, you are ready to go on to the second step of the nursing process: *diagnosis*. This step is an important one because this is when you will *analyze the data to identify the nursing diagnoses and problems that will be the basis of your plan of care*. You *must* identify the problems before you can plan for nursing care. This chapter first gives an overview of the state of the art of nursing diagnosis, and then discusses the actual how-to's of problem identification.

* Carpenito L: Personal communication, October 26, 1985

The Evolution of Nursing Diagnoses

For two decades, nurses have been struggling to define the term "nursing diagnoses." Both the American Nurses' Association (ANA) *Standards for Nursing Practice* (1973) and the ANA *Social Policy Statement* (1980) encourage nurses to use nursing diagnoses in their practice. However, there has been much controversy over what problems are and what problems are not nursing diagnoses.

In an effort to help identify categories of problems that should be considered to be nursing diagnoses, a group of nurses met in 1973 to form the National Conference Group for the Classification of Nursing Diagnoses. This group, made up of theorists, educators, administrators, and practitioners has since become the North American Nursing Diagnosis Association (NANDA). As a result of the group's work, NANDA has published a list of nursing diagnoses that have been accepted for testing and study. The list, which appears in Display 3-1, has become widely accepted for use in identifying nursing diagnoses.

Display 3-1.   *Nursing Diagnoses Approved by the North American Nursing Diagnoses Association*

Activity Intolerance

Activity Intolerance, Potential

Adjustment, Impaired*

Airway Clearance, Ineffective

Anxiety

Body Temperature, Potential Alteration in*

Bowel Elimination, Alteration in: Constipation

Bowel Elimination, Alteration in: Diarrhea

Bowel Elimination, Alteration in: Incontinence

Breathing Pattern, Ineffective

Cardiac Output, Alteration in: Decreased

Comfort, Alteration in: Pain

Comfort, Alteration in: Chronic Pain*

Communication, Impaired: Verbal

Coping, Family: Potential for Growth

Coping, Ineffective Family: Compromised

Coping, Ineffective Family: Disabling

Coping, Ineffective Individual

Diversional Activity, Deficit

Family Process, Alteration in

Fear

Fluid Volume, Alteration in: Excess

Fluid Volume Deficit, Actual

Fluid Volume Deficit, Potential

Gas Exchange, Impaired

Grieving, Anticipatory

Grieving, Dysfunctional

Growth and Development, Altered*

Health Maintenance, Alteration in

Home Maintenance Management, Impaired

Hopelessness*

Hyperthermia*

Hypothermia*

(continued)

Display 3-1 *(Continued)*

Incontinence, Functional*

Incontinence, Reflex*

Incontinence, Stress*

Incontinence, Total*

Incontinence, Urge

Infection, Potential for*

Injury, Potential for: (poisoning, potential for; suffocation, potential for; trauma, potential for)

Knowledge Deficit (specify)

Mobility, Impaired Physical

Neglect, Unilateral*

Noncompliance (specify)

Nutrition, Alteration in: Less than Body Requirements

Nutrition, Alteration in: More than Body Requirements

Nutrition, Alteration in: Potential for More than Body Requirements

Oral Mucous Membrane, Alteration in

Parenting, Alteration in: Actual

Parenting, Alteration in: Potential

Post Trauma Response*

Powerlessness

Rape Trauma Syndrome

Self-Care Deficit: feeding, bathing/hygiene, dressing/grooming, toileting

Self-Concept, Disturbance in body image, self-esteem, role performance, personal identity

Sensory-Perceptual Alteration: visual, auditory, kinesthetic, gustatory, tactile, olfactory

Sexual Dysfunction

Sexuality Patterns, Altered*

Skin Integrity, Impairment of: Actual

Skin Integrity, Impairment of: Potential

Sleep Pattern Disturbance

Social Interaction, Impaired*

Social Isolation

Spiritual Distress (distress of the human spirit)

Swallowing, Impaired*

Thermoregulation, Ineffective*

Thought Processes, Alteration in

Tissue Integrity, Impaired*

Tissue Perfusion, Alteration in: cerebral, cardiopulmonary, renal, gastrointestinal, peripheral

Urinary Elimination, Alteration in Patterns

Urinary Retention*

Violence, Potential for: self-directed or directed at others

* diagnoses approved for study in 1986

Carpenito (1985 c) suggests that nurses are involved with treating two types of problems: *nursing diagnoses* and *collaborative* problems.

Nursing diagnoses are problems that can be prevented, resolved, or reduced through *independent* nursing interventions. Independent nursing interventions are those nursing actions that are encompassed by licensure and law and that require no supervision or direction by others (Potter and Perry, 1985). Some examples of independent nursing interventions are assisting with activities of daily living, patient teaching, and promoting mobility. *Collaborative problems* are problems that can be prevented, resolved, or reduced through *collaborative* or *interdependent* nursing interventions. Interdependent nursing interventions are nursing actions that can be legally performed only under the direction of a licensed, qualified professional (often a physician).

The above definitions of nursing diagnoses and collaborative problems are broad descriptions, and we must define the terms more specifically if we are fully to understand what they mean. Let's take a look at how nursing diagnoses and collaborative problems are defined in specific terms.

Defining Nursing Diagnoses

Gordon describes a nursing diagnosis as an "actual or potential health problem that nurses, by virtue of their education and experience, are capable and licensed to treat" (Gordon, 1976). Shoemaker describes a nursing diagnosis as being a "clinical judgment about an individual, family or group which is derived through a deliberate, systematic process of data collection and analysis" (Shoemaker, 1985). Carpenito suggests that nursing diagnoses may also be used to label health states or interaction patterns of individuals or groups (Carpenito, 1985 c). Keeping all these definitions in mind, this book will define nursing diagnosis as follows:

> *Nursing diagnosis:* An actual or potential health problem (of an individual, family, or group) that nurses can legally treat independently, initiating the nursing interventions necessary to prevent, resolve, or reduce the problem

Nursing diagnoses are statements of an individual's or group's *human response* to their health state and are often described as an actual or potential alteration in health. Because the human response is greatly influenced by each person's *own unique perspective*, the use of nursing diagnoses requires nurses to seek to view health management through the eyes of the individual. For example, a physician may perform an interview and physical examination and conclude that the individual is in good health. However, a nurse may perform a similar interview and exam and identify some nursing diagnoses because the person, himself, perceives that he is not in good health or could be in better health. Nursing diagnoses often describe health problems that include how the person as a whole feels. This includes determining how well *determined how* the person is functioning as a total human being, including the physical, psychological, sociocultural, developmental, and spiritual aspects of life. For example, consider how a nurse and a physician may present the same information to a given patient:

> *Physician:*   "All your lab work is complete, and I'm happy to tell you that you are in very good health."
>
> *Nurse:*   All your lab work is complete, and I'm happy to tell you that physically you seem to be in good health. . . . Do you *feel* as if you are in good health? . . . How is everything going?"

For clarification of the types of problems that nursing diagnoses describe, study the NANDA-accepted list of nursing diagnoses in Display 3-1.

Defining Collaborative Problems

Carpenito defines a collaborative problem as being an "actual or potential problem that may occur as a result of complications of disease, diagnostic studies, or treatments and that can be prevented, resolved, or reduced by interdependent, or collaborative, nursing interventions."* This book will support this definition for collaborative problems.

> *Collaborative problem:* An actual or potential problem that may occur from complications of disease, diagnostic studies, or medical or surgical treatment, and that can be prevented, resolved, or reduced through collaborative nursing interventions

To clarify, look at Figure 3-1, which shows some examples of potential complications that may arise as a result of disease, treatments, or diagnostic studies.

Writing Diagnostic Statements for Collaborative Problems

Because collaborative problems deal with potential complications, it is suggested that you use the term "potential complication" to describe the problem.* For example, if you are working with an intravenous line, you may identify the problem of "potential complication: phlebitis." Using the words "potential complication" helps you focus your nursing assessment for that specific complication. For instance, if you use the "intravenous line" example, the collaborative problem of "potential complication: phlebitis" would

---

* Carpenito L: Personal communication, October 26, 1985

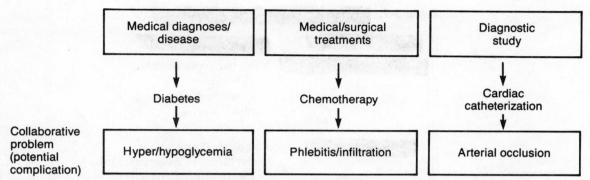

Figure 3-1. *This chart shows an example of a possible potential complication (collaborative problem) resulting from disease, medical or surgical treatment, or diagnostic studies.*

direct you to assess for signs of phlebitis (pain, redness, swelling) at the site of the intravenous line insertion. Using the words "potential complication" will also help you to be more specific about the collaborative problem. If you simply said "collaborative problem: intravenous line," you would not be clear as to exactly what the problem might be. Using "potential complication" gives a clearer description of the problem.

Table 3-1 (page 62) shows some examples of collaborative problems that nurses who work in an acute care setting frequently encounter.

Differentiating Nursing Diagnoses from Collaborative Problems

Differentiating nursing diagnoses from collaborative problems is important because you must be aware of what problems can be treated by independent nursing interventions and what problems necessitate collaboration with other health-care professionals. Using the term "nursing diagnosis" to label those health problems that nurses can treat independently will encourage nurses to initiate independent nursing interventions and to begin to research those activities that should be implemented independently for specific nursing diagnoses. On the other hand, using the term "collaborative problem" will help nurses to focus on collaborative interventions and the collaborative nursing role. Including both nursing diagnoses and collaborative problems in your plan of care will help you to focus on all aspects of nursing care. It will help reduce the possibility of your tending to focus only on either your collaborative role or only on your independent role as a nurse.

Table 3-1. *Common Collaborative Problems*

Source of Problem	Collaborative Problem
Intravenous therapy	Potential complications: Phlebitis IV infiltration Fluid overload Infection
Nasogastric suction	Potential complications: Occlusion of nasogastric tube Electrolyte imbalance
Skeletal traction	Potential complication: Poor alignment of bones
Medications	Potential complications: Side-effects Adverse reaction/allergy Overdosage
Foley catheter	Potential complications: Blockage of the catheter Infection
Chest tubes	Potential complications: Blockage of the chest tube Hemo/pneumothorax Infection Bleeding
Surgery	Potential complications: Bleeding Electrolyte imbalance Respiratory difficulties Infection Oliguria/anuria Shock/hypovolemia Fluid overload/congestive heart failure Nausea/vomiting

The following diagram illustrates the difference between nursing diagnoses and collaborative problems.

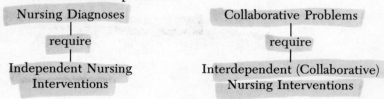

Nursing Diagnoses

require

Independent Nursing
Interventions

Collaborative Problems

require

Interdependent (Collaborative)
Nursing Interventions

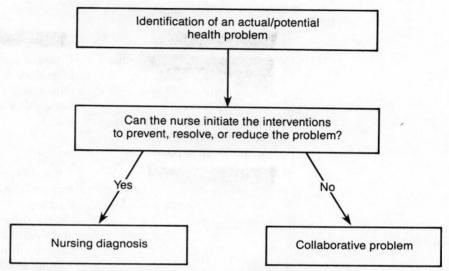

Figure 3-2. *Differentiation between a nursing diagnosis and a collaborative problem.*

Each time that you identify an actual or potential problem, you must ask yourself, "Can I initiate the treatments necessary to prevent, resolve, or reduce this problem *independently?* If the answer is "yes," then you have identified a nursing diagnosis. If the answer is "no," then you *must* seek direction from the appropriate health-care professional. To clarify the difference between a nursing diagnosis and a collaborative problem, look at Figure 3-2.

For further clarification, look at the examples of nursing diagnoses and collaborative problems listed in Display 3-2.

Display 3-2. *Examples of Nursing Diagnoses and Collaborative Problems*

Nursing Diagnosis	**Collaborative Problem**
(Nurse treats independently)	(Nurse collaborates)
Ineffective Airway Clearance related to poor positioning (Nurse repositions patient independently.)	Potential complication: hypoxemia secondary to pneumonia (Nurse collaborates with physician regarding treatment regimen—e.g., antibiotics, oxygen.)

(continued)

Display 3-2. *(Continued)*

Nursing Diagnosis	**Collaborative Problem**
Impairment of Skin Integrity related to immobility (Nurse turns and repositions patient to prevent pressure points and keeps skin clean and dry. These actions are initiated independently.)	Potential complication: evisceration secondary to wound dehiscence (Nurse collaborates with physician to establish a regimen for wound care.)
Knowledge Deficit: Self-administration of insulin (Nurse implements a teaching plan independently.)	Potential complication: dehydration/ malnutrition secondary to tube feedings (Nurse collaborates with physician and dietitian to establish type and amount of tube feedings to be administered.)

Table 3-2 shows how a given patient in a given situation or with a given medical diagnosis is likely to have both collaborative problems and nursing diagnoses that need nursing care.

Table 3-2

Situation/Medical Diagnosis	Nursing Diagnosis	Collaborative Problem
Pneumonia	Potential Fluid Volume deficit related to insufficient fluid intake	Potential complication: hypoxemia
Prescribed bed rest	Potential Impairment of Skin Integrity related to prescribed bed rest	Potential complication: hemostasis/thrombus formation
Diabetes	Knowledge Deficit: Insulin therapy	Potential complication: hyper/hypoglycemia
Insertion of chest tubes	Impaired Physical Mobility related to pain and presence of chest tubes	Potential complication: hemo/pneumothorax

Figure 3-3 shows the diagnostic process beginning with assessment and culminating with formulation of nursing diagnoses and collaborative problems.

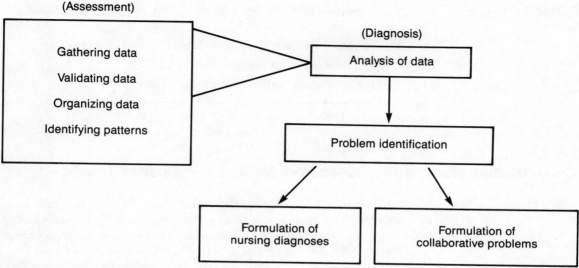

Figure 3-3. *The diagnostic process.*

☐ *Practice Session* *Nursing Diagnoses/Collaborative Problems*
(suggested answers on page 164)

For each of the following problems, write ND in front of the ones that are nursing diagnoses and CP in front of the ones that are collaborative problems. (For each problem, ask yourself, "Can the nurse independently initiate the major interventions for this problem?" If the answer is "yes," label it ND. If the answer is "no," label it CP.)

1. *CP* Potential complication: hemorrhage
2. *ND* Potential Ineffective Airway Clearance related to copious secretions
3. *ND* Potential for Injury related to generalized weakness
4. *CP* Potential complication: fluid volume overload secondary to intravenous therapy
5. *ND* Fluid Volume Deficit related to insufficient fluid intake
6. *ND* Alteration in Skin Integrity related to pressure points
7. *CP* Potential complication: cardiac arrhythmias
8. *CP* Potential complication: septicemia
9. *ND* Diversional Activity Deficit related to prescribed bed rest
10. *CP* Potential complication: increased intracranial pressure
11. *CP* Potential complication: malnutrition secondary to prescribed NPO

(continued)

12. _CP_ Alteration in Nutrition: Less than body requirements related to poor appetite

13. _ND_ Impaired Physical Mobility related to prescribed bed rest

14. _CP_ Potential complication: pneumothorax

15. _CP_ Potential complication: thrombus formation

Differentiating Nursing Diagnoses from Medical Diagnoses

Medical diagnoses focus on identifying diseases, while nursing diagnoses focus on identifying human responses and alterations in the person's ability to function as an independent human being. For example, two people may have the same disease but may have very different responses to the disease. Consider the cases of Mr. Smith and Mr. Jones below:

Case History I

Mr. Smith has had the medical diagnosis of diabetes for 5 years. He is knowledgeable about his disease and manages his own insulin injections and diet very well.

Case History II

Mr. Jones has just (last week) been diagnosed as having diabetes. He says that he is depressed because he hates being sick and is afraid of having to give himself his own injections.

Both people have the same medical diagnosis with very different human reactions that will identify very different nursing diagnoses (*e.g.*, Mr. Jones will have the nursing diagnosis of *Fear related to having to give himself his own injections,* but this nursing diagnosis is inappropriate for Mr. Smith even though he, too, has the medical diagnosis of diabetes). Table 3-3 compares nursing diagnoses and medical diagnoses.

Working with the NANDA List of Nursing Diagnoses

The NANDA list (Display 3-1) is the result of many nurses working together to refine and label nursing diagnostic categories so that they can be used by all nurses. This work of refining nursing diagnoses is in its beginning stages. There is a long way to go, but nurses *do have a beginning*. Nursing is beginning to label what it is that nursing knows and does. The NANDA list

Table 3-3. *Comparison of Medical Diagnoses and Nursing Diagnoses*

Medical Diagnosis	*Nursing Diagnosis*
Describes a disease	Describes a human response
Stays the same as long as the disease is present	May change from day to day as human reactions change
Treatable by physicians within the scope of medical practice	Treatable by nurses within the scope of nursing practice
Often deals with actual patho-physiologic changes within the body	Often deals with the *patient's perception* of his own health state
Applies to diseases in individuals only	May apply to alterations in individuals or groups

is not without faults—it may be incomplete and unrefined, but it is a beginning, and nurses across the country are using many of these diagnoses to provide a basis for nursing care. It is important to continue to work with the NANDA list for several reasons:

☐ Using a nationally accepted list of diagnoses will help nurses to communicate with each other using common terminology. Nursing knowledge will be easier to learn and teach if authors, faculty, and clinicians all use the same terminology. (Imagine if physicians could use any word they wanted to describe pneumonia!)

☐ Using common terminology will facilitate the use of computers for nursing. (Nurses will be able to retrieve records according to nursing diagnoses rather than medical diagnoses, and therefore will be able to collect data to further research in nursing.)

☐ Using a nationally accepted list of diagnostic categories provides a method for reimbursement according to nursing activities related to nursing diagnoses rather than just medical diagnoses.

☐ All nurses can work together toward testing and refining the diagnostic categories to identify assessment criteria and nursing interventions that nurses can use to improve nursing care.

This chapter focuses on identifying nursing diagnoses both by using the NANDA-accepted list and by generating your own specific nursing diagnoses. It is this author's philosophy that *if you can use NANDA terminology to define the nursing diagnosis, you should use their terms.* If you cannot find a diagnosis on the list that accurately describes the health problem that you have identified, then write your own nursing diagnosis using the guidelines set forth in this chapter.*

Components of the NANDA Diagnostic Category Labels

Each of the category labels for nursing diagnoses accepted by NANDA consists of three components:

1. Title (or label)
2. Defining characteristics (signs and symptoms)
3. Etiological and contributing factors

Display 3-3 further describes the components of each diagnostic category.

Display 3-3.   *Diagnostic Category Components*

Title (or label): Offers a concise description of the health problem

Defining characteristics: Cluster of signs and symptoms that are often seen with that particular diagnosis

Etiological and contributing factors: Identifies those situational, pathophysiological, and maturational factors that can cause or contribute to the problem

Display 3-4 shows the specific diagnostic components for the diagnostic category of *Alteration in Bowel Elimination: Constipation.*

Display 3-4.   *Diagnostic Category Components for Alteration in Bowel Elimination: Constipation*

Title (or Label)

Alteration in Bowel Elimination: Constipation

* It should be noted that both Gordon (1982 b) and Carpenito (1984 a) have described additional nursing diagnoses that are not on the official NANDA list of accepted diagnoses as of November 1985. For those who wish to submit a nursing diagnostic label for study by NANDA, guidelines for submitting a nursing diagnosis can be found in the appendix.

Display 3-4   (Continued)

Defining Characteristics

Hard, formed stool

Decreased bowel sounds

Defecation occurs less than three times a week

Reported feeling of rectal fullness

Reported feeling of pressure in rectum

Straining and pain on defecation

Palpable impaction

Etiological and Contributing Factors

Pathophysiological

Malnutrition

Sensory/motor disorders

  Spinal cord lesions

  Spinal cord injury

  Cerebrovascular accident (stroke)

  Neurological diseases

Drug side-effects

  Antacids

  Iron

  Barium

  Aluminum

  Calcium

  Anticholinergics

  Anesthetics

  Narcotics (codeine, morphine)

Metabolic and endocrine disorders

  Anorexia nervosa

  Obesity

  Hypothyroidism

  Hyperparathyroidism

Pain (upon defecation)

  Hemorrhoids

  Back injury

Decreased peristalsis related to hypoxia (cardiac, pulmonary)

Situational

Surgery

Lack of exercise

Irregular evacuation patterns

Dehydration

Habitual laxative use

Fear of rectal or cardiac pain

Lack of privacy

Inadequate diet (lack of roughage/thiamine)

Maturational

Infant: Formula

Child: Toilet training (reluctance to interrupt play)

Elderly: Decreased motility of GI tract

(From Carpenito L: Handbook of Nursing Diagnosis, pp 8–9. Philadelphia, JB Lippincott, 1984)

The PES Format

Recognizing the importance of having all three components in a nursing diagnostic label (problem, etiology, and signs and symptoms), Gordon (1976) has suggested the PES format for describing nursing diagnoses to confirm, or validate, the presence of a nursing diagnosis. Display 3-5 describes the PES format.

Display 3-5. *Gordon's Suggested PES Format for Validating Nursing Diagnoses*

To describe the diagnosis, incorporate the following:

1. State the problem (P).
2. State the etiology (E) using "related to."
3. State the signs and symptoms (S) using "as manifested by."

Example I: Powerlessness related to hospitalization

P—Powerlessness

E—related to hospitalization

S—as manifested by the patient verbalizing that he feels angry and depressed that he can do nothing to change the fact that he has to be hospitalized

Writing Diagnostic Statements for Actual Nursing Diagnoses

When you write a diagnostic statement for an actual nursing diagnosis, you should use Gordon's PES system to describe the diagnosis* and write a three-part statement that includes the following:

1. The problem (P)
2. Its cause or etiology (E)
3. The signs and symptoms (defining characteristics) that are evident in the patient (S)

Most authors recommend that you use the phrase *"related to"* to link the problem and its etiology together (*e.g.*, *Impaired Verbal Communication*

* Carpenito L: Personal communication, 1985

related to complete deafness). The phrase *"as manifested by"* is added to describe the signs and symptoms, or defining characteristics, that are evident. For example, you would write "Impaired Verbal Communication *related to* complete deafness, *as manifested by* inability to follow verbal instructions and inability to talk." When you identify an actual nursing diagnosis, it is important to be sure that you write all three parts of the statement so that the diagnosis is confirmed by stating the signs and symptoms that are present in this specific patient. Display 3-6 summarizes the components of a three-part statement for actual nursing diagnoses.

Display 3-6. *Three-Part Diagnostic Statement for Actual Nursing Diagnoses*

1. Health problem: Ineffective Airway Clearance
                                            ↓
                                       related to
                                            ↓

2. Etiology: weak cough and incisional pain
                                            ↓
                                    as manifested by
                                            ↓

3. Signs and symptoms: poor or no cough effort and statements
   (defining characteristics) that incision hurts too much when he
                              coughs

Diagnostic statement: Ineffective Airway Clearance related to weak cough and incisional pain, as manifested by poor or no cough effort and statements that incision hurts too much when he coughs

---

☐ *Practice Session*   *Using the PES Format to Validate Actual Nursing Diagnoses*
                          (*suggested answers on page 164*)

Read all of the data for each of the case histories below and write a three-part diagnostic statement that clearly describes the diagnosis.

(*continued*)

☐ *Practice Session*

1. Mr. Starr has the following signs and symptoms:

   Chronic cough productive of mucus

   States he has smoked three packs of cigarettes a day for 15 years

   Smokes constantly in his room

   Elevated arterial CO_2

   You identify the diagnosis of Impaired Gas Exchange.

2. Bob O'Brien has the following signs and symptoms:

   States he has had no appetite for 2 weeks

   You have recorded a 10-lb weight loss.

   He weighs 15 lb less than his recommended weight.

   You identify the diagnosis of Alteration in Nutrition: Less Than Body Requirements.

3. Lilly Johns has the following signs and symptoms:

   She is unable to move either leg.

   She has limited passive range of motion in lower joints.

   You identify the diagnosis of Impaired Physical Mobility.

4. Mr. Bell has the following signs and symptoms:

   Mr. Bell is blind.

   He states he falls and bumps himself often.

   He states he gets confused as to where things are when he is away from the familiarity of his home.

   He has a large bruise over his right forehead which he says he got when he bumped himself on an open cabinet door.

   You identify the diagnosis of Potential for Injury.

Writing Diagnostic Statements for Potential and Possible Nursing Diagnoses

It is as important to identify *potential* and *possible* nursing diagnoses as it is to identify *actual* nursing diagnoses. If you identify a potential nursing diagnosis before it actually occurs, you can take measures to prevent its occurrence. If you identify a possible nursing diagnosis, you alert everyone to learn more about the patient to determine if the patient actually does have the nursing diagnosis. Identifying possible diagnoses helps to ensure that all the problems that could be present are considered in determining the plan of care.

So, you may ask, "How do I know when there is a potential or possible nursing diagnosis?"

If you assess your patient and note that there are some high-risk factors present that may cause him to have a certain nursing diagnosis, then you have identified a potential nursing diagnosis. (Carpenito, 1985b) For example, suppose you were taking care of an elderly woman who was very thin, immobile, and bedridden. She may have had excellent care at home, and as a result has beautiful, healthy looking skin. However, you should be aware that her age, weight, immobility, and confinement to bed can be contributing or etiological factors for *Impairment of Skin Integrity*. You should then document the potential nursing diagnosis by writing a two-part statement that describes both the problem and its cause* (*e.g., Potential Impairment of Skin Integrity related to advanced age, immobility, and confinement to bed*). You would then establish a plan of nursing care that would prevent her from getting irritated or broken skin (*e.g.,* establish a regimen of frequent assessment of pressure points, such as the coccyx, and of frequent turning, repositioning, and massaging to promote circulation to the skin).

You may find that sometimes you may suspect that a patient may have a specific nursing diagnosis because of some cues that *may seem* to suggest a possible problem. For example, during your initial nursing assessment of a client who has been admitted with cancer, he may have stated that he didn't believe in God—that he did at one time, but not anymore. This sort of statement may suggest the *possible* diagnosis of *Spiritual Distress,* or it may simply mean that his beliefs have changed during the course of his life. You would then document the diagnosis by writing a two-part statement that describes both the problem and its cause* (*e.g., Possible Spiritual Distress related to current illness*). Your plan of nursing care for this possible diagnosis would be to gather more data to determine if the client actually does have *Spiritual Distress* (*e.g.,* plan to spend time discussing what the patient believed in the past and the factors that have changed his beliefs). Identifying a *possible* diagnosis is important because it will help you to focus your

* Carpenito L: Personal communication, October 1985

ongoing data collection to confirm or negate the presence of the nursing diagnosis.

When you are analyzing patient data, it is important that you consider actual, potential, and possible nursing diagnoses because all three should be considered when planning comprehensive nursing care. When you identify an *actual* nursing diagnosis, you should always use a three-part statement (using *"related to"* and *"as manifested by"*) to confirm the diagnosis. When you identify a *potential* or *possible* diagnosis, you should use a two-part statement using *"related to"* and eliminating the *"as manifested by"* because there are no *clear* signs and symptoms to be described. Display 3-7 summarizes how to write two-part and three-part diagnostic statements.

Display 3-7. *Writing Two-Part and Three-Part Diagnostic Statements*

1. Actual nursing diagnosis (three-part statement):

   | Problem + Etiology + Signs and symptoms present |

   EXAMPLE:

   Self-care Deficit related to inability to move both arms as manifested by casts on both hands and wrists

2. Potential and possible nursing diagnoses (two-part statement)

   | Problem + Etiology |

   EXAMPLES:

   Potential Ineffective Airway Clearance related to smoking

   Possible Disturbance in Self-concept related to chronic illness

Comparison of Actual, Potential, and Possible Nursing Diagnoses

Study Table 3-4, which compares actual, potential, and possible nursing diagnoses.

Table 3-4. *Comparison of Actual, Potential, and Possible Nursing Diagnoses*

Nursing Diagnosis	Signs and Symptoms Present?	Etiological/ Contributing Factors Present?	Nursing Plan
Actual nursing diagnosis	Yes	Yes	Monitor signs and symptoms present to determine improvements or deterioration in condition.
			Identify interventions to reduce or eliminate the cause of the problem.

Table 3-4 *(Continued)*

Nursing Diagnosis	Signs and Symptoms Present?	Etiological/ Contributing Factors Present?	Nursing Plan
Potential nursing diagnosis	No	Yes	Perform daily focus assessments to determine if signs and symptoms have appeared to change status from *potential* to *actual*. Identify interventions to prevent, reduce, or remove contributing factors.
Possible nursing diagnosis	Unsure	Unsure	Gather more data to clarify vague cues and to determine if the signs and symptoms or contributing factors are actually present.

(Adapted with permission from Carpenito L: Unpublished workshop notes, 1985)

☐ *Practice Session*   *Writing Diagnostic Statements for Potential and Possible Nursing Diagnoses*
(suggested answers on page 165)

Read the data for each of the case histories below and write a two-part diagnostic statement that clearly describes the diagnosis.

1. Mr. Reardon has been confined to bed with casts on both his legs. He seems angry and has stated that he does not want to talk to anyone. You are aware that he has had a fight with his girlfriend. You suspect that he may have the diagnosis of *Ineffective Individual Coping related to confinement to bed or possibly problems with significant others.* However, you are not sure if Mr. Reardon's withdrawal is a temporary method of coping that works for him.

   NURSING DIAGNOSIS:

2. Mr. Cappelli has a temperature of 101° F. He sleeps a lot and has a poor appetite. He drinks about 2000 ml a day if you offer frequent fluids and encourage him to drink. You recognize that fever is a contributing factor for *Fluid Volume Deficit.*

   NURSING DIAGNOSIS:

(continued)

□ *Practice Session*

3. Mr. Rogers has just had his gallbladder removed today under general anesthesia. His nursing assessment form has documented that he has smoked a pack of cigarettes a day for the past 20 years. He has no productive cough at present, but you recognize that his smoking and recent general anesthesia are contributing factors for *Ineffective Airway Clearance*.

NURSING DIAGNOSIS:

4. You see Mrs. Jackson in clinic 6 weeks after a hysterectomy. She states that she feels well physically, but that emotionally, she just doesn't feel like herself yet. She states that she gets angry easily and cries a lot. She states that she feels that she gets no support from her husband. You note that her nursing assessment form from her admission to the hospital for the hysterectomy 6 weeks ago recorded that she had expressed concern about the effect of hysterectomies on sexual functions. You suspect that she may have the diagnosis of *Sexual Dysfunction*.

NURSING DIAGNOSIS:

Using Nursing Diagnosis Terminology

Learning how to write diagnostic statements that clearly define both the problem and its etiology can be difficult at first. The following guidelines are suggested to help prevent errors:

□ *Guidelines*   *How to Prevent Errors When Writing Diagnostic Statements*

□ Don't state the nursing diagnosis in medical terminology.

EXAMPLE:

Incorrect: Mastectomy related to cancer

Correct: Potential Alteration in Self-concept related to loss of right breast

□ Don't state the nursing diagnosis as a medical diagnosis.

☐ *Guidelines*

EXAMPLE:

Incorrect: Potential for pneumonia

Correct: Ineffective Airway Clearance related to poor cough effort

☐ Don't state the nursing diagnosis as a nursing intervention.

EXAMPLE:

Incorrect: Offer the bedpan frequently related to urinary urgency

Correct: Alteration in Urinary Elimination related to urinary urgency

☐ Don't write the nursing diagnosis as a nursing problem.

EXAMPLE:

Incorrect: Noncompliance for whirlpool treatments related to pain

Correct: Alteration in Comfort: Pain related to whirlpool treatments

☐ Don't be vague. Be specific.

EXAMPLE:

Incorrect: Ineffective Airway Clearance related to difficulty breathing

Correct: Ineffective Airway Clearance related to incisional pain

☐ Don't write a nursing diagnosis which repeats a physician's order.

EXAMPLE:

Incorrect: NPO (Nothing by mouth)

Correct: Alterations in Oral Mucosa related to order of NPO

☐ Do not state two problems at the same time.

EXAMPLE:

Incorrect: Pain and Fear related to diagnostic procedures

Correct: Fear related to unfamiliarity with diagnostic procedures
Alteration in Comfort: Pain related to diagnostic procedures

☐ Don't write the diagnostic statement in such a way that it may be legally incriminating.

EXAMPLE:

Incorrect: Potential for Injury related to lack of siderails on bed

Correct: Potential for Injury related to disorientation

☐ Don't "rename" a medical problem to make it a nursing diagnosis (Carpenito, 1985c).

EXAMPLE:

Incorrect: Alteration in Hemodynamics related to hypovolemia

Correct: Hypovolemia (This is a medical problem and should be stated as such.)

(*continued*)

☐ *Guidelines* ☐ Don't write a nursing diagnosis based on value judgments.

EXAMPLE:

Incorrect: Spiritual Distress related to atheism as manifested by statements that he has never believed in God

Correct: There may be no diagnosis in this situation. The person may be at peace with his beliefs.

☐ *Practice Session* **Identifying Correctly Stated Nursing Diagnoses**
(suggested answers to page 165)

For each of the nursing diagnostic statements listed below, put C in front of the ones that are correctly stated.

1. _____ Alteration in Bowel Elimination related to cancer

2. _____ Potential for malnutrition

3. _____ Potential for pneumonia

4. _____ Need for increased fluids related to thirst

5. _C_ Ineffective Individual Coping related to sensory bombardment

6. _C_ Potential Fluid Volume Deficit related to fever and sore throat

7. _____ Lung cancer related to metastasis

8. _C_ Alteration in Self-concept related to mastectomy

9. _____ Anxiety related to unknown etiology

10. _____ Infection related to burns

11. _____ Alteration in Communication

12. _____ Sudden Infant Death Syndrome related to low birth weight

13. _C_ Potential for Violence related to inability to vent anger

14. _C_ Alteration in Urinary Elimination related to Foley catheter

15. _C_ Alteration in Urinary Elimination related to bedwetting

---

The Process of Identifying Nursing Diagnoses

Now that we discussed how nursing diagnoses should be clearly stated, let's take a look at how nursing diagnoses can be identified.

In order to learn to identify nursing diagnoses, it is important to learn how to identify health problems in general. You will find that different nurses will use different approaches to identifying problems. Some will systematically test for the presence of several different possible problems, and others will very quickly identify the problems present with minimal questioning. *The speed and accuracy of problem identification will depend on each nurse's skill and knowledge.* Beginning nurses and nursing students must develop strategies that help to ensure the most accurate identification of problems. The following guidelines are suggested to assist you in developing strategies for identifying health problems.

□ *Guidelines*

Identifying Health Problems/Nursing Diagnoses

1. Determine what is the usual and present pattern of behavior/health for the client. Then identify health-care needs that are not being met.

    Is there a problem with breathing or circulation?

    Is there a problem with nutrition or elimination?

    Is there a problem with fluid intake/output?

    Is there a problem with injury or disease?

    Is there a problem with safety?

    Is there a problem with rest or exercise?

    Is there a problem with the person's ability to think or to perceive his environment?

    Is there a psychological, developmental, spiritual, or sociocultural problem?

    Is there a role/relationship problem?

2. Ask the client (and family) what he views as problems for himself. Identify these as problems.

3. To clearly identify the exact nature of the problems, be aware of the "do's" and "do not's" of problem identification:

    Do not overvalue the probability of one explanation for a problem.

    Do explore alternative possibilities that further explain the problem.

    Do not maintain a narrow focus and fail to consider all pertinent data.

    Do keep an open mind. Be aware of your own biases when making inferences about the data that you have gathered.

    Do not jump to conclusions.

    Do take your time to avoid hasty interpretations that may not be correct.

Using Nursing Literature to Help Analyze Health Problems

Very few nurses are experts at everything. Some nurses are very knowledgeable in certain areas, but most nurses recognize the need to continue to grow in knowledge and expertise. As a professional, you must acknowledge the necessity of utilizing appropriate nursing journals, texts, and audiovisuals to learn about the data that you have obtained about your patient. For example, suppose that you have gathered the information that your patient is a diabetic and you know very little about the disease. It would be your responsibility as a nurse to read and learn about the disease, its effects on the body, its possible complications, and its common treatments before you could adequately identify actual and potential problems. Reviewing pertinent literature is a valuable activity that can greatly add to your ability to analyze data and identify health problems.

Identifying Usual Life-styles and Coping Patterns

Another aspect of identifying the exact nature of a health problem or nursing diagnosis is that of identifying usual life-styles and coping patterns. In order to fully understand how a given problem might be affecting a specific individual's sense of well-being, it is necessary to consider how the person spends his days. For example, a person who must be on his feet all day would probably consider a painful foot to be a bigger problem than a person who is able to spend some time sitting with his foot up on a pillow. Learning about a person's life-style may also help to identify some factors that are actually contributing to the problem. For example, you may find out that a person who has chronic constipation hates to exercise and lives an exceedingly sedentary life, which could contribute to the constipation.

Identifying how a person usually copes with changes in life-style helps to determine how the person might be able to deal with the health problem. For example, a person who likes to do physical exercise or work when he is depressed may find confinement to a bed more difficult than a person who simply likes to read to get his mind off his problems.

Determining the Etiology of Nursing Diagnoses/Problems

As stated earlier, nursing diagnoses are described by stating both the problem and its causative factors, or etiology. Therefore, in many ways, it is as important to learn how to identify the etiology of a problem as it is to identify the problem itself.

Just as with problem identification, identifying etiologies depends on the individual nurse's nursing knowledge, experience, and analytical skills. Learning to identify etiologies will become easier as you grow in theoretical and technical nursing knowledge. However, there are some questions that you can ask to help in identifying etiologies of health problems. Consider the questions listed in Display 3-8.

Display 3-8.   *Questions for Identifying the Etiology
of a Health Problem*

What are the factors that the client (or family) identify as causing or contributing to the problem?

Are there factors related to developmental age, presence of disease, or situational changes in life-style that could be contributing to the problem?*

Have your other resources for data collection/analysis (medical records, other health-care professionals, literature review) identified some factors that might be causing or contributing to the problem?

What factors do you yourself feel might be causing or contributing to the problem?

* Carpenito (1983) offers common etiological contributing factors for each nursing diagnostic category according to situational, pathophysiological, and maturational factors.

The role of etiological and contributing factors in determining *specific* nursing interventions will be discussed in Chapter 4, Planning.

Identifying Nursing Diagnoses on the NANDA List

The NANDA list of accepted categories of nursing diagnoses provides assistance to nurses who are learning to label nursing diagnoses. You should become familiar with this list and learn the definition, defining characteristics, and common etiologies for each category. Learning more than 50 category labels may seem to be an insurmountable task, but it *will* become easier as you work with each of the categories. The following guidelines are suggested to help you to learn how to identify when your patient has a nursing diagnosis that is on the accepted NANDA list.

☐ *Guidelines*   *Learning How to Identify NANDA-Accepted Nursing Diagnoses*

☐ Become familiar with the list.

1. To help you learn the category labels, their defining characteristics, and common etiologies, carry a handbook that contains this information in a quick-reference format.*

* Recommended: Carpenito LJ: Handbook of Nursing Diagnoses. Philadelphia, JB Lippincott, 1984. This book contains the category labels, defining characteristics, and common etiologies. It also correlates medical diagnoses with the common nursing diagnoses.

(continued)

☐ *Guidelines*

2. Study the list and choose some diagnoses that you feel you will encounter frequently, and learn these first. For example, *Alteration in Bowel Elimination, Potential Impaired Skin Integrity, Fear,* and *Anxiety* are diagnoses that even beginning nursing students are able to identify.

3. Do not feel that you have to use every diagnosis on the list. If you are philosophically opposed to using a certain diagnosis, throw that diagnosis out, but not the entire list.

☐ Follow the steps for identifying nursing diagnoses/problems.

1. Practice using focus assessment tools that help to gather specific data for each particular diagnosis.*

2. Gather, interpret, and cluster your signs and symptoms (objective and subjective data).

3. Be aware of medical diagnoses present because certain nursing diagnoses are frequently associated with certain medical diagnoses (*e.g.*, people with diabetes have a high potential for Impairment of Skin Integrity).

4. Study the signs and symptoms that you have clustered together, and choose a diagnostic label that seems to describe the problem. *Compare the signs and symptoms with the defining characteristics for that particular diagnostic category.* All of the defining characteristics need not be present, but at least one should be evident in order to confirm the diagnosis.

5. Be specific when you use an accepted diagnostic label. Use qualifying or quantifying adjectives to clearly identify the diagnosis (*e.g., Potential Impairment of Skin Integrity related to complete loss of sensation and mobility of lower half of body*).

6. If the diagnostic category is followed by the word "specify," this means you should use a colon and specify the area where the problem occurs. For example, if you identify *Knowledge Deficit,* you must specify in what area the person needs to learn (*e.g., Knowledge Deficit: Side-effects of medications*).

7. Remember, a nursing diagnosis should reflect a *pattern in responses,* not a response that happens just one time.

Identifying Nursing Diagnoses That Are Not on the NANDA List

The NANDA list of nursing diagnoses is incomplete. Therefore, you may find that you identify a problem that you feel should be considered to be a nursing

---

* Specific focus assessment criteria questions for each nursing diagnosis category can be found in Carpenito LJ: Nursing Diagnosis: Application to Clinical Practice. Philadelphia, JB Lippincott, 1983.

diagnosis, and yet you may not be able to find a category label on the list that describes it appropriately. The following guidelines are suggested for labeling a nursing diagnosis that is not on the accepted list.

□ *Guidelines*

Identifying Nursing Diagnoses Not on the NANDA List

1. Gather, interpret, and cluster your signs and symptoms (objective and subjective data).
2. Be sure that you are not renaming a medical diagnosis or problem. If it's a medical problem, call it a medical problem. (For example, call hypotension by its own name. Don't rename it "alteration in hemodynamics.")
3. Be sure that you haven't made any of the common errors for stating nursing diagnoses (See Guidelines for Helping to Prevent Errors When Writing Diagnostic Statements).
4. Be sure that none of the NANDA category labels are appropriate to describe the problem.
5. State the problem and its etiology and list the defining characteristics for this particular patient using the PES format, if possible.

   EXAMPLE:

   Destructive Behavior related to poor role model at home as manifested by playing with matches and abusing school property

---

□ *Key Points*

Analyzing Data to Identify Nursing Diagnoses and Collaborative Problems

1. Diagnosis involves analyzing assessment data to identify actual and potential nursing diagnoses and collaborative problems.
2. As a professional, you must acknowledge the necessity of using appropriate nursing journals, audiovisuals, and texts to learn about the data you have gathered about your patient.
3. Nursing diagnoses differ from collaborative problems in that they can be treated by nursing interventions that are *independent*, while collaborative problems require *interdependent* nursing interventions.
4. Each of the diagnoses listed by NANDA has three components:

   The category label (problem)

   The defining characteristics (cluster of signs and symptoms often seen with the diagnosis)

   The common etiologies for the problem

(*continued*)

5. You should use NANDA terminology to describe the diagnoses that you have identified whenever possible. However, if you diagnose a health problem that can be treated independently, but cannot find a category label on the NANDA list that adequately describes this problem, you should write the nursing diagnosis in your own terms, using the PES format.

6. When writing a diagnostic statement for *actual* nursing diagnoses, you should write a three-part statement using the PES format.

   EXAMPLE:

   Impaired Verbal Communication related to inability to speak English as manifested by inability to follow instructions in English and verbalizing requests in Spanish

7. When writing a diagnostic statement for a *potential* or *possible* nursing diagnosis, you should write a two-part statement that describes both the problem and its etiology.

   EXAMPLES:

   Potential for Fear related to bad previous experience of being left alone at night

   Possible Knowledge Deficit: Colostomy care

8. When writing a problem statement for a collaborative problem you should use the word "potential complication" to clearly describe the collaborative problem.

   EXAMPLES:

   Potential complication: hypoxemia secondary to pneumonia

   Potential complication: infection secondary to central venous line

9. To adequately analyze the effect of a given problem on a given person, the person's usual life-style and methods of coping must be considered.

10. The following guidelines can be found in this chapter for review:

    Guidelines to prevent making errors when writing diagnostic statements

    Guidelines for identifying health problems/nursing diagnoses

    Questions for identifying the etiology of a health problem

    Strategies to help you learn how to identify nursing diagnoses that are on the NANDA-accepted list

    Guidelines for identifying nursing diagnoses that are not on the NANDA list

☐ *Practice Session*   *Identifying Nursing Diagnoses and Collaborative Problems*
(*suggested answers on page 165*)

Study the data given for each of the following case histories. Identify cues, make inferences about the cues, and on a separate piece of paper list the nursing diagnoses and collaborative problems that you can identify (actual, potential, possible). Use the PES format to validate your diagnoses.

Case History I   (Mrs. Goode, 31 years old)

Medical Diagnosis
Cerebral concussion

Subjective Data

States she was hit on the head by a falling branch

States she has a headache and feels dizzy when she lifts her head off the pillow

Expressed concern about having her husband look after her two children because "he is not good with them"

States she is afraid of hospitals and needles

States she has never worked outside the home because her children need her

States "I can't stay in bed and use the bedpan as the doctor said"

Objective Data
Age: 31; Ht: 5'3"; Wt: 160 lb

Nursing Physical Assessment

Temperature: 98.4°F

Pulse: 78 and regular

Respirations: 24 and nonlabored

Blood Pressure: 128/72

Moves all extremities with equal strength

Pupils are equally reactive to light.

Large bruise over right forehead

Abdomen soft, nontender, obese

Peripheral pulses strong

IV in right arm looks red and infiltrated.

Case History II   (Mr. Northe, 54 years old)

Medical Diagnosis
Atrial fibrillation/rule out myocardial infarction

Subjective Data

States this is his second "heart attack"

(*continued*)

□ *Practice Session*

States that he is "worried about being in bed for 3 weeks like last time"

Complains of mild chest discomfort in the substernal area, says "it feels like gas"

Says he is glad he has good insurance for his wife and family—his brother, who was only 2 years older, died of a heart attack last year

Complains of having had no appetite for 3 days, and that he hasn't had a bowel movement in 5 days

States he hates being on bed rest because he gets "stiff all over from not moving"

Objective Data
Age: 54; Ht: 5'11"; Wt: 160 lb

Nursing Physical Assessment

Temperature: 97.8°F

Pulse: 64 and irregular (monitor shows atrial fibrillation without PVCs)

Respirations: 32

Blood Pressure: 140/92

Skin: warm, dry, and pink

Lungs: a few scattered rales at bases

Oxygen on at 4 liters/min via cannula

Becomes easily short of breath

Peripheral pulses satisfactory

IV with potassium in left arm at 100 ml/hr

Intake last 24 hours = 2400 ml

Output last 24 hours = 1000 ml

Note two red pressure areas on both heels

□ *Bibliography*

American Nurses' Association: Nursing: A Social Policy Statement. Kansas City, MO, American Nurses' Association, 1980

American Nurses' Association: Standards of Nursing Practice. Kansas City, MO, American Nurses' Association, 1973

Aspinall M: Nursing diagnosis—The weak link. Nurs Outlook 24: 433–437, 1976

Aspinall M, Tanner C: Decision-Making for Patient Care: Applying the Nursing Process. New York, Appleton-Century-Crofts, 1981

Bates B: A Guide to Physical Examination, 3rd ed. Philadelphia, JB Lippincott, 1983

Berger M: Clinical thinking ability and nursing students. Journal of Nursing Education 23(7): 306–308, 1984

Carnevali D: Nursing Care Planning: Diagnosis and Management. Philadelphia, JB Lippincott, 1983

Carnevali D, Mitchell P, Woods N, Tanner C: Diagnostic Reasoning in Nursing. Philadelphia, JB Lippincott, 1984

Carpenito L: Nursing Diagnosis: Application to Clinical Practice. Philadelphia, JB Lippincott, 1983

Carpenito L: Handbook of Nursing Diagnosis. Philadelphia, JB Lippincott, 1984 a

Carpenito L: Is the problem a nursing diagnosis? Am J Nurs 84(11):1418–1419, 1984 b

Carpenito L: Diagnosing nutrition problems. Am J Nurs 85(5): 584, 1985 a

Carpenito L: Diagnostics: Actual, potential, or possible nursing diagnoses. Am J Nurs 85(4):458, 1985 b

Carpenito L: Nursing diagnosis: Selected dilemmas in practice. Occupational Health Nursing. August:397–400, 1985 c

Gordon M: Nursing diagnosis and the diagnostic process. Am J Nurs 76:1298–1300, 1976

Gordon M: Nursing Diagnosis: Process and Application. New York, McGraw-Hill, 1982 a

Gordon M: Manual of Nursing Diagnosis. New York, McGraw-Hill, 1982 b

Griffith J, Christensen P: Nursing Process: Application of Theories, Frameworks and Models. St Louis, CV Mosby, 1982

Kozier B, Erb G: Fundamentals of Nursing: Concepts and Process. Menlo Park, CA, Addison-Wesley, 1979

Kim MJ, McFarland GK, McLane AM: Classification of Nursing Diagnosis: Proceedings of the Fifth National Conferences. St Louis, CV Mosby, 1984

Leslie FM: Nursing diagnosis use in long-term care. Am J Nurs 81:1012–1014, 1981

Potter P, Perry A: Fundamentals of Nursing Concepts: Concepts, Process, and Practice. St Louis, CV Mosby, 1985

Price M: How nursing diagnosis helps focus your care: The patient is starving... but why. RN 42:45–48, 1979

Price M: Nursing diagnosis: Making a concept come alive. Am J Nurs 80:668–671, 1980

Shoemaker J: Characteristics of a nursing diagnosis. Occupational Health Nursing 33:387–389, 1985

Sjoberg EL: Nursing diagnosis and the COPD patient. Am J Nurs 83:245–248, 1983

☑ Setting priorities
☑ Establishing goals
☑ Determining nursing interventions
☑ Documenting the plan of care

4
Planning

Standard III: *The plan of nursing care includes goals derived from the nursing diagnoses.*

Standard IV: *The plan of nursing care includes priorities and the prescribed nursing approaches or measures to achieve the goals derived from nursing diagnoses.*

Standard V: *Nursing actions provide for client/patient participation in health promotion, maintenance, and restoration.*

Standard VI: *Nursing actions assist the client/patient to maximize his health capabilities.* *

*Abstracted from Standards—Nursing Practice. Copyright American Nurses' Association, 1973

□ *Glossary*

Care plan, patient   A written plan of nursing care that describes specific client problems, expected outcomes, nursing orders, and client progress

Client outcome (or client goal, or client objective)   A statement of a behavior that would demonstrate the improvement or resolution of a specific problem described by the identified nursing diagnoses or collaborative problems

Etiology   Factors that cause or contribute to a problem

Long-term goal   An objective that is expected to be achieved over a relatively long period of time, usually weeks or months

Measurable verb   Verbs that describe an exact behavior that you can *see* or *hear*

Nursing goal   A statement of what the nurse plans to do to help the client achieve an expected outcome (*e.g.,* "to teach Bobby how to give an injection") or of her own personal objectives (*e.g.,* "to attend inservice on stress reduction")

Nursing intervention (nursing action)   An activity performed by the nurse and the client to prevent illness (or its complications) and to promote, maintain, or restore health

Nursing order   A statement written by the nurse that specifies nursing interventions that all nurses caring for that specific patient should follow

Nursing standard   A statement of how a nurse should give nursing care in a certain situation. Nursing standards are determined by the law, the ANA, and each individual health-care facility

POMR (Problem-oriented medical records)   A method of documenting a patient's care whereby all health-care professionals caring for a given patient chart the identified problems in the same place, using SOAP format

Short-term goal   A goal that is expected to be achieved in a relatively short period of time, usually less than a week

SOAP charting   A method of documenting a plan of care by charting the following data:

    S = Subjective data

    O = Objective data

    A = Assessment (problem statement)

    P = Plan (goals)

SOAPIE charting   A method of documenting a plan of care by charting the following data

    S = Subjective data

    O = Objective data

    A = Assessment (problem statement)

    P = Plan (goals)

    I = Interventions

    E = Evaluation

Once you have identified specific nursing diagnoses and collaborative problems for an individual patient or client, you are ready to begin the third step of the nursing process: *planning*. This is the time when you will determine how to give nursing care in an organized, individualized, goal-directed manner. Planning will involve the following:

☐ Setting priorities

☐ Establishing client goals/expected outcomes

☐ Determining nursing actions/intervention

☐ Documenting the plan of nursing care

Setting Priorities

More than ever, today's nurse must learn how to set priorities. This is a time when health-care agencies are working to cut costs. Many nurses are finding themselves working with sicker and sicker patients and less and less help. As a nurse, it will not be unusual for you to find yourself with twenty wonderful things you could do for your patient and only time to perform five or ten. It will be important that you know which are the five or ten most important things—you will have to learn to assess a situation and set priorities.

When providing nursing care for individuals, families, or groups, you will find that problems, situations, and priorities can change from day to day and hour to hour. You will have to learn to be flexible and set priorities according to the current status of the situations and problems present. Most authors suggest that the first step in setting priorities is that of making a list of the problems (nursing diagnoses and collaborative problems) that you have identified during assessment. You then must study the list and decide which are the most important problems.

Next, you will have to decide the order of nursing care (*i.e.*, what problems you will look after first). You will not always resolve one problem before another. More often you will be working on several different problems during the course of the day, making some progress on each one. For example, you may diagnose the problem of *Alteration in Nutrition: Less Than Body Requirements*. You may also be working on the problems of *Impaired Physical Mobility* and *Powerlessness*. You will probably be working on all of these problems at different times during the day, and will make some progress on each one but not necessarily resolve one before the other. However, you must ask yourself whether one problem is contributing to another. For example, you may be trying to teach a person how to give his own insulin injection and find that he is not receptive. Perhaps he has a problem of denial and actually is denying he has diabetes. In this case, the problem of denial should be dealt with before the problem of not knowing how to give an injection.

The questions in Display 4-1 are suggested to help you set priorities.

Display 4-1. *Questions to Ask When Setting Priorities*

1. Which are the problems that *must* be taken care of immediately (*e.g.*, life-threatening problems)?

2. Which are the problems that you will work to prevent, reduce, or resolve today?

3. Is there a relationship between any of the problems that necessitates one being resolved before another can be resolved? (*i.e.*, Is one problem causing or contributing to another?)

4. Of the problems you will work on today, which will you work on first . . . second . . . third . . . ?

5. Are there any problems that can be worked on at the same time? (For example, you may choose to work on promoting communication about fears and concerns about illness while assisting the client with morning care.)

6. Which of the problems should be addressed on the nursing care plan? (Only the problems that are unique, unusual, or complex should be addressed on the nursing care plan. For example, if you have diagnosed the problem of *Fluid Volume Deficit related to dislike of drinking fluids,* you should address this problem by giving specifics of the types of fluids the person likes and exactly how many milliliters the person should drink during each shift. Routine care problems, such as meeting routine requirements of daily hygiene, should not be addressed unless there is a unique problem.)

☐ *Guidelines*   *Setting Priorities*

☐ Applying Maslow's hierarchy of basic needs, the problems can be given the following order of priority:

Priority #1: Problems interfering with physiological needs (*e.g.*, problems with respiration, circulation, nutrition, hydration, elimination, temperature regulation, physical comfort)

Priority #2: Problems interfering with safety and security (*e.g.*, environmental hazards, fear)

Priority #3: Problems interfering with love and belonging (*e.g.*, isolation or loss of a loved one)

Priority #4: Problems interfering with self-esteem (*e.g.*, inability to wash hair, perform normal activities)

☐ *Guidelines*   *Priority #5:* Problems interfering with the ability to achieve personal goals

☐ Priority ratings will be influenced by the following:

The client's own perception of priorities: Ask the person what he feels is important, and explain your rationale if you have to impose a different set of priorities.

The overall treatment plan: For example, you may plan to have the person eat earlier than usual on the days he has a physical therapy treatment.

The overall health status of the client: For example, *Knowledge Deficit* may be given a high priority rating for a newly diagnosed diabetic if the person is generally healthy. However, this same problem would be given a low priority if the patient was too ill to learn.

The presence of potential problems: For example, assisting a patient to stand immediately postoperatively to reduce the potential of falling takes priority over the patient's desire to stand on his own.

Giving Goal-Directed Care

Establishing goals is a necessary part of the planning phase of the nursing process because it is important to be sure that everyone knows what is to be accomplished and when it is expected to be accomplished. For example, if a nurse tells her patient, "By tomorrow, I expect that you'll be able to demonstrate how to give an injection," he knows that he must practice today until he is competent in giving an injection. Knowing that today is the last day for practice will motivate him. The nurse will also know that today is the last day for practice and will be motivated to spend time helping the patient practice. Both the client and the nurse are more likely to meet with success the next day because the goal was clear. Setting goals with your clients will help to reduce misunderstandings about the plan of care and give incentive to both the client and you.

Short-Term and Long-Term Goals

Giving goal-directed care includes setting both long-term and short-term goals. Short-term goals (STG) are those that can be met relatively quickly, often in less than a week. Long-term goals (LTG) are those that are to be achieved over a longer period of time, often weeks or months. Frequently, a nurse may set several short-term goals in order to reach a long-term goal. Display 4-2 gives some examples of short-term goals that may be stepping stones to a long-term goal.

Display 4-2. *Examples of Short- and Long-Term Goals*

Short-Term Goal	**Long-Term Goal**
"Mrs. Smith will demonstrate how to hold her newborn infant by tomorrow (6/9)."	"Mrs. Smith will demonstrate how to dress, feed, and bathe her newborn infant by discharge (6/13)."
"Mrs. Fox will turn and re-position herself from side to side every 2 hours."	"Mrs. Fox will maintain good skin integrity while she is on bed rest."
"Mr. Roberts will demonstrate how to change his colostomy bag within 2 days (by 7/7)."	"Mr. Roberts will demonstrate how to give complete colostomy care according to hospital standards by discharge (by 7/21)."
"Susie will walk with crutches with assistance by 3 days after surgery (by 7/28)."	"Susie will walk unassisted with a cane by discharge (by 8/10)."

Long-term goals may also include goals that are ongoing (*i.e.*, goals that are to be accomplished every day). These types of long-term goals are usually stated by using the words "every day" or "will maintain." Note the examples below:

☐ "Louise will dress herself every morning."
☐ "Mr. Nathaniel will maintain a fluid intake of 2000 ml a day."

Many agencies use the abbreviation "LTG" to describe the *overall goal* of the plan of care. This type of long-term goal is also considered to be the "discharge goal" for the client. These long-term goals, or discharge goals, should be clearly stated on the care plan so that the whole team knows that "this is what we are all working toward." For example, you may be caring for two women who are both in their seventies and have had surgery for a fractured hip. One of them may have an LTG of "returns to her husband and home, independently ambulatory with cane, capable of performing her usual activities of daily living," while the other woman's LTG may read "returns to nursing home and continued complete bed rest with healed fracture, good leg alignment, and without complications." Writing overall LTGs on the care plan is important so everyone who contributes to carrying out the plan is realistic and clear concerning what they expect the plan of care to accomplish.

Nursing Goals versus Client Goals

During the planning phase, nurses are involved with setting both their clients' goals (client outcomes) and their own goals (nursing goals). The client goal describes what the nurse expects that her client will be able to accomplish. The nursing goal describes what the nurse expects to do in order to help the client accomplish the client goal. For example, a *client goal* may be "will demonstrate safe crutch walking." The corresponding *nursing goal* for this client goal would be "to teach the client how to walk with crutches."

On a given day, nursing goals may also include the nurse's own individual objective for learning. For example, a student may have goals of nursing care for a new mother on a maternity floor and have a separate personal learning goal of "observing two deliveries." Both of these goals are legitimate nursing goals and should be considered when the nurse plans activities for the day. However, your personal learning objectives should not impede nursing care for your patient. You must plan ahead so that your own goals can be met and your client still receives good nursing care.

Client goals are usually clearly stated on the care plan so that everyone is aware of what the client is aiming to do. On the other hand, nursing goals are usually formulated mentally and are only stated when someone asks, "What are your goals and activities for today/tomorrow?"

Study Display 4-3 which shows the relationship between client goals and nursing goals.

Display 4-3. *Comparison of Nursing Goals and Client Goals*

Nursing Goal	Client Goal
Describes how the nurse hopes to accomplish the client goal. (*e.g.*, "Teach Mr. Jones how to use crutches safely by 6/1.")	Describes what the client is expected to accomplish as a result of the nursing goals (*e.g.*, "Mr. Jones will demonstrate safe crutch walking by 6/1.")
Gives direction to selecting nursing activities (*i.e.*, What must the nurse do to accomplish the goal of nursing care?)	Gives direction to client activities. (*i.e.*, What must the client do to accomplish his goal?)
May include the nurse's own personal objectives for learning	Includes only client-oriented objectives
Usually formulated mentally	Clearly documented on the nursing care plan

Display 4-4 lists nursing goals with corresponding client goals.

Display 4-4. *Example Nursing Goal with Corresponding Client Goal*

Nursing Goal	Client Goal
"To teach Mrs. Rose how to use a walker without assistance by Saturday (8/1)"	"Mrs. Rose will walk unassisted with a walker by Saturday (8/1)"
"To maintain good hygiene for Mr. Jones"	"Mr. Jones will be clean shaven, bathed, and have good oral hygiene every day."
"To prevent skin breakdown on the elbow area of Mrs. Hayes"	"Mrs. Hayes will have no sign of skin irritation on her elbows."

Establishing Client Goals (Client Outcomes)

When you establish expected client outcomes, you establish the goals or objectives that you have decided will demonstrate an improvement or resolution of your client's problems (*i.e.*, the nursing diagnoses and collaborative problems that you identified during the assessment phase). The terms "outcomes," "objectives," and "goals" are often used interchangeably because they all are a statement of what is expected to be accomplished by the plan of care. Client goals describe what the client will be able to do by a specific time.

Describing both what the client will be expected to accomplish and by when he will be able to accomplish it serves two purposes:

☐ Both the client and the nurse know what has to be accomplished when in order to reduce or resolve the identified problems.

☐ The established goal, or outcome, can later be studied to evaluate how well the plan of care is working (*i.e.*, has the goal been met?).

Display 4-5 lists several examples of expected outcomes (or client goals or objectives).

Display 4-5. *Examples of Expected Outcomes/Client Goals*

"Mr. James will stop smoking by November 11."

"Ms. Michaels will lose 5 lb in 3 weeks (by July 31)."

"Mrs. Matthews will walk unassisted with crutches by February 6."

"Mr. Daniels will demonstrate sterile injection technique by September 18."

Expected outcomes are derived from the nursing diagnoses and collaborative problems that you have identified during the analysis (diagnosis) phase of the nursing process. *For each nursing diagnosis or collaborative problem that you have identified on the nursing care plan, you must formulate a specific client outcome, or goal.* If your diagnoses are not correct, then it is unlikely that your goals will be appropriate for the patient.

The client outcome (or goal) for a given problem is a statement of a patient behavior that would demonstrate an improvement in, or resolution of, the problem. For example, you may have identified the nursing diagnosis of *Potential Ineffective Airway Clearance.* An acceptable outcome or goal for this diagnosis might be "the patient will maintain a clear airway."

Display 4-6 shows the steps a nurse should take in establishing outcomes.

Display 4-6. *Steps for Deriving Outcomes from Nursing Diagnoses/Problems*

1. Look at the first clause of the nursing diagnosis or problem statement (*i.e.,* the word or words before "related to").

First Clause

Example: ⎡Potential Impairment of Skin Integrity⎤
related to immobility

2. Now restate the first clause in a goal statement that would describe an improvement in or absence of the problem.

Example: The client will demonstrate no signs of skin irritation or breakdown.

Display 4-7 lists several examples of outcomes that are derived from nursing diagnoses and collaborative problems that have been identified during a nursing assessment.

Display 4-7. *Client Outcomes (Goals) Derived from Nursing Diagnoses/Collaborative Problems*

Nursing Diagnosis/Collaborative Problem	**Corresponding Client Outcome (Goal)**
Potential Impairment of Skin Integrity related to confinement to bed	Client will demonstrate no signs of skin irritation or breakdown.

(continued)

Display 4-7. *(Continued)*

Alteration in Nutrition: Less Than Body Requirement related to poor eating habits	Client will eat three healthy meals with two fruit snacks daily.
Potential complication: wound evisceration 2° to open surgical wound	Wound will remain intact (will be protected by special non-allergenic dry dressing and elastic binder when ambulating).

Sometimes you will find that you decide to write more than one goal for a given problem. In these cases, the goals will probably relate to the etiology of the problem rather than to the problem itself. It is important that *at least one* of the goals ensure that the problem described in the problem statement is improved. Note the following example:

☐ *Nursing Diagnosis: Alteration in Nutrition: More Than Body Requirements related to poor eating habits and minimal physical activity*

   Goal #1: Client will describe daily menus that demonstrate healthy meal choices and decreased intake of empty calories. (This goal relates to the problem of "poor eating habits," which is a causative factor.)

   Goal #2: Client will attend daily exercise classes. (This goal relates to the problem of "minimal physical activity," which is a causative factor.)

   Goal #3: Client will lose 1 lb per week beginning 10/25 until she weighs between 135 and 145 lb. (This goal demonstrates a *direct resolution* of the problem of *Alteration in Nutrition: Less Than Body Requirements.*)

Be sure that at least one of the goals that you set demonstrates a direct resolution of the problem statement.

Applying Nursing Standards When Setting Client Goals

When you are establishing outcomes, it is necessary to apply accepted standards of nursing care (*i.e.,* your outcomes and plan of nursing care must reflect that you have set forth a plan that will achieve acceptable standards of care). Standards of care will be determined by the following:

☐ *The Law:* Nurse Practice Acts differ from state to state. You must be aware of your individual state practice acts, which delineate the scope of nursing and the ways in which nurses should practice.

☐ *The American Nurses' Association (ANA):* The ANA has established standards that should be applied in all areas of nursing practice. They have also set standards for the specialty areas (*e.g.,* maternity, community health, rehabilitation).

☐ *The Institution:* Each institution usually evolves its own unique set of standards that reflect the values and beliefs of the system (*i.e.,* the institution decides what objectives must be met in order to demonstrate optimum nursing care and then decides what interventions are necessary to accomplish the objectives). These objectives and interventions then become the standards that are set down in the policies and procedure manuals of the institution.

When you are setting client goals and planning nursing care you must apply the standards that are set forth by the law, the ANA, and the institution where you are working. ANA standards apply to all nurses everywhere and are applied throughout your nursing education. Individual state laws and institutional policies and procedures differ, so you must make yourself responsible for learning these as you move from institution to institution (*i.e.*, be sure to read policy and procedures manuals and become familiar with your state practice act).

Some health-care agencies will have established outcome criteria for certain problems. In other words, they have recorded (either in their computer or in their procedure manual) the outcomes or goals that they feel would demonstrate a high standard of achievement for a patient with a certain problem. For example, a hospital may list in its procedure book that the outcome criteria for a patient who has undergone an appendectomy should be the following:

☐ Will ambulate the first day after the appendectomy
☐ Will be free from postoperative complications during the first 2 days of surgery (*i.e.*, no bleeding, no respiratory problems, no signs of infection)
☐ Will demonstrate how to change his dressing the third day after surgery
☐ Will verbalize how to observe incision for healing or infection by the third day after surgery
☐ Will be discharged free of complications with written instructions for self-care on the fourth day after the appendectomy

Ideally these types of outcomes are designed to maximize health care. However, other factors, such as cost containment, may influence the determination of what is considered to be an outcome that demonstrates high-quality care. Therefore, it is extremely important that nurses become intimately involved in the development of these criteria.

If the agency where you are working has established certain outcome criteria for certain situations or problems, then you should use them as a guide to help you to establish your own client goals. For example, using the example of the person with an appendectomy, you should refer to the outcome criteria listed under Appendectomy, and, if appropriate, you should make these outcomes your goals. If you identify more problems, you should add more outcomes or goals. For example, you may identify the additional problem of *Potential Ineffective Individual Coping related to extreme dislike for having activity restrictions as manifested by statements of concern about not being able to cope with restrictions.* You would then add the outcome or goal of *will verbalize methods of coping with the stress of activity restrictions by discharge.*

When you are working within an institution, it is important to be aware of any established outcome criteria because these are the goals or outcomes that will be used to evaluate whether the plan that you have set forth for the patient was successful. If the goals that you have set forth are not congruent with the goals or outcome criteria established by the institution, then you are not likely to succeed in the eyes of the institution.

Rules for Stating Client Outcomes/Goals/Objectives

Client outcomes must be specific. They must not only state *what* is to be done, but also *who* is to do it, *when* they are to do it, *how* and *where* they are to do it, and *how well* they are to do it. To ensure that outcomes are specific, there are rules for writing outcome statements. Each goal or outcome statement must have the components listed in Display 4-8 below.

Display 4-8. *Components of Goal Statements/Expected Outcomes*

1. *Subject: Who* is the person expected to achieve the goal?
2. *Verb: What actions* must the person do to achieve the goal?
3. *Condition: Under what circumstances* is the person to perform the actions?
4. *Criteria: How well* is the person to perform the action?
5. *Specific time: When* is the person expected to perform the action?

   Example: Mr. Smith will walk with a cane at least to the end of the hall and back this afternoon.

Subject: Mr. Smith

Verb: will walk

Condition: with a cane

Criteria: at least to the end of the hall and back

Time: this afternoon.

Making sure that the goal statement has all five of these components ensures a very specific outcome that can later be evaluated to see how well the patient has achieved the goal that you have set for him.

"Fine Tuning" Outcome Statements.   Because client outcomes deal with describing exactly what a patient must be able to *do,* it is important that clear and specific verbs are used to describe *what is to be done.* For example, a nurse who wants the patient to understand how to use sterile technique may be tempted to write an outcome of "The patient will understand how to use sterile technique." However, this outcome would be too vague. You must ask yourself, "*How* will I *know* if he understands?" The only way that you can be sure if he does indeed understand is if he actually verbalizes or demonstrates how to use sterile technique. Verbs used in writing outcomes must be verbs that are *measurable* (*i.e.*, verbs that describe the exact behavior that you expect to *see* or *hear*). Below are some examples of verbs that are measurable and verbs that are nonmeasurable. *When writing client outcomes, avoid using the verbs listed in the nonmeasurable columns.*

Display 4-9. *Examples of Measurable and Nonmeasurable Verbs*

Measurable Verbs

identify	perform	exercise
describe	demonstrate	communicate
perform	share	cough
relate	express	walk
state	has an increase in	stand
list	has a decrease in	sit
verbalize	has an absence of	discuss

Non-measurable Verbs

know	think
understand	accept
appreciate	feel

There are many things to consider when establishing goals. The following guidelines are suggested to help you set goals for your clients.

□ *Guidelines*   *Establishing Goals/Outcomes*

□ Be realistic in establishing goals—be sure to consider the following:

   Growth and development

   Behavioral patterns of the individual

   Physical health state

   Available human and material resources

   Other planned therapies for the client

   The time frame in which the client may be expected to achieve an expected outcome

(continued)

□ *Guidelines*

□ Whenever possible, set goals mutually with the client and others involved in his health care (*e.g.*, family, other health-care workers) to ensure that the goals are congruent with other planned therapies.

□ Establish both short- and long-term goals (the short-term goals can be used as steps toward meeting the long-term goal).

□ Be sure that the client goals that you write describe a client behavior or action that demonstrates the desired improvement or resolution of the problems identified by the nursing diagnoses or collaborative problems listed on the nursing care plan.

□ Follow the rules for writing goal statements.

□ Use measurable, observable verbs to describe the desired actions or behaviors that you expect to see (Display 4-9).

□ Identify only one behavior per outcome. If you need to write two behaviors, write two outcomes.

EXAMPLE:

> *Wrong:* Client will discuss the role of insulin in carbohydrate metabolism and give his own insulin.
>
> *Right:* Client will discuss the role of insulin in carbohydrate metabolism.
> Client will give his own insulin.

□ Be sure that the subject of your outcome statement is the client (or family) or some part of the client.

EXAMPLES:

> *Bob* will rest lying down for a half hour after meals.
> The *skin* around the incision will remain clean and dry at all times.

□ Be sure that your outcomes reflect the accepted standards of the ANA, your state practice act, and the institution where you are working.

□ *Practice Session*

Writing Expected Goals/Outcomes
(suggested answers on page 166)

1. List at least five measurable verbs.

2. Choose the client goal statements that are written correctly below. Identify what is wrong with the statements that are written incorrectly.
a. John will know the basic four food groups by 1/4.

□ *Practice Session*   b. Mrs. Smith will demonstrate how to use her walker by Saturday.

c. Mr. Jones will (improve) his appetite by 1/6.

d. Jane will list the equipment needed to change sterile dressings by 2/2.

e. Susan will walk independently in the hall after surgery.

f. Mrs. Baylis will understand the importance of maintaining a salt-free diet. *by when?*

g. June will ambulate to the bathroom with the use of her cane by 3/4.

h. Mrs. Smith will appreciate the importance of childproofing her home. *by when*

i. Janet will lose 5 lb by 1/9.

j. Mr. Collins will feel less pain by Thursday.

□ *Practice Session*   *Establishing Client Goals/Expected Outcomes*
(suggested answers on page 166)

For each diagnosis or problem below, write an appropriate client outcome. Be sure that each client outcome that you write has all of the necessary components. (See Display 4-8, "Components of Goal Statements/Expected Outcomes," if you need help.)

1. Potential Alteration in Bowel Elimination: Constipation related to poor roughage intake in diet

2. Alteration in Oral Mucous Membrane related to poor oral hygiene

3. Potential Impairment in Skin Integrity related to draining abdominal incision

4. Impaired Verbal Communication related to inability to speak English

5. Spiritual Distress related to inability to attend daily Mass

6. Self-Care Deficit: Feeding, related to weakness of both hands

7. Potential Ineffective Airway Clearance related to smoking

☐ *Practice Session*   8. Alteration in Nutrition: Less Than Body Requirements related to loss of appetite

9. Sleep Pattern Disturbance related to need for frequent treatments and assessment of vital signs

10. Alteration in Patterns of Urinary Elimination related to urinary urgency

---

Affective, Cognitive, and Psychomotor Outcomes/Objectives

Expected outcomes can be classified into three domains: cognitive, affective, and psychomotor. Below is a description of each of the domains.

☐ *Cognitive domain:* Outcomes that are associated with acquired knowledge or intellectual abilities (*e.g.*, learning the signs and symptoms of diabetic shock)

☐ *Psychomotor domain:* Outcomes that deal with developing motor skills (*e.g.*, mastering how to walk with crutches)

☐ *Affective domain:* Outcomes that are associated with changes in attitudes, feelings, or values (*e.g.*, deciding that old eating habits need to be changed)

Display 4-10 lists verbs that are representative of each domain.

Display 4-10. *Verbs Representative of the Three Domains*

Cognitive	Affective	Psychomotor
teach	express	demonstrate
discuss	share	practice
identify	listen	perform
describe	communicate	walk
list	relate	administer
explore	value	give

Correctly identifying the domains of the client outcomes is an important aspect of planning nursing strategies. Many beginning nurses assume that the only strategies that are necessary are those that promote new knowledge or skills and forget to be concerned with the need for a new set of values. For example, it could be useless to instruct a client how to stick to a diabetic diet if he did not value the importance of being on the diet in the first place. Often more than one domain may be involved in the achievement of one outcome. For example, you may have identified the expected outcome of "Mrs. Laird will prepare three balanced meals for her children." In order to achieve this outcome, Mrs. Laird will have to achieve outcomes in all three domains. She will have to:

☐ State the foods that should be included in a balanced diet (cognitive)

☐ Share her feelings concerning being responsible for her children's nutrition (affective)

☐ Demonstrate cooking and serving the meal (psychomotor)

☐ *Practice Session*   *Domains of Expected Outcomes*
(suggested answers on page 167)

1. Identify whether each of the expected outcomes listed below is in the affective, cognitive, or psychomotor domain. (Remember, there may be more than one domain for each outcome.)

   a. Mrs. Resh will demonstrate how to prepare and sterilize her baby's formula.

   b. Becky will discuss the importance of sterilization.

   c. Judy will relate her feelings concerning going home.

   d. Mrs. Ballard will discuss the relationship between blood sugar levels and food.

   e. Connie will administer her own insulin according to the results of her morning blood sugar readings.

   f. Mr. Roberts will walk the length of the hall with a cane.

   g. Mrs. Bell will verbalize when she is worried or concerned.

   h. Debbie will demonstrate how to perform postural drainage.

   i. Matt will verbalize the signs and symptoms of hypoglycemia.

   j. Jimmy will eat a balanced breakfast every morning.

2. Once you have identified the domains of the expected outcomes in the above examples, write one or two activities that would help the client to achieve the outcome. (Note the example below.)

   EXAMPLE:

   Sample outcome: Mrs. Jones will be able to dress herself without assistance by 7/4.

☐ *Practice Session*   *Domain:* Psychomotor

Activities: Practice buttoning buttons and tying shoes on 7/1 and 7/2. Practice putting on blouse, skirt, shoes, and socks on 7/3. Demonstrate dressing herself on 7/4.

Determining Nursing Interventions for Nursing Diagnoses

Broadly speaking, the aim of nursing interventions should be

☐ To promote health

☐ To maintain health

☐ To restore health

☐ To prevent complications

☐ To provide for optimum physical, psychological, and spiritual comfort

In order to provide for comfort, to prevent complications, and to promote, maintain, or restore health, nurses must use a variety of interventions. The activities listed below are all nursing interventions that nurses are likely to identify when planning for comprehensive nursing care.

☐ Performing nursing assessments to identify new problems and to determine the status of existing problems

☐ Performing patient teaching to help clients gain new knowledge concerning their own health

☐ Counseling clients to make decisions about their own health care

☐ Consulting with and referring to other health-care professionals to obtain appropriate direction

☐ Performing specific treatment actions to remove, reduce, or resolve health problems

☐ Assisting clients to perform activities themselves

Let's consider the nurse's role of assessing, teaching, counseling, and consulting when providing for patient care.

Nursing Assessment as an Intervention

Performing a focus assessment of identified problems is a common nursing intervention that should be employed before performing any intervention. You must assess the status of the problem before you begin to intervene. For example, if you use the example diagnosis of *Fluid Volume Deficit related to insufficient fluid intake,* you must assess how much the person has actually had to drink before you encourage him to drink more. It could be possible that he has overcompensated and is now drinking more than he should.

Blindly continuing nursing interventions without performing a focus assessment of the problem can create new problems and be detrimental to the individual's health.

Teaching as an Intervention

Teaching is an intervention that is common to many problems. It may be a specific intervention (such as teaching an individual to give his own injection) or it may be an adjunct intervention (such as explaining the rationale for coughing and deep breathing while you are assisting the patient to cough and deep breathe). Teaching is a vital nursing intervention that should be implemented at every opportunity. The following guidelines are suggested to help you in planning patient teaching.

□ *Guidelines*   *Planning Patient Teaching*

□ Always assess readiness to learn and previous knowledge before you begin a teaching plan.

□ Set goals with the client so that both of you know what you are aiming to teach (*e.g.*, "Let's see if by this afternoon you can describe menus that would contain three balanced meals").

□ Use terminology that the client understands.

□ Encourage the client to ask questions and verbalize his understanding of what is being taught (*e.g.*, by stating, "I want you to feel free to ask questions no matter how stupid you think they are. We all feel dumb from time to time, so don't feel you are the only one. Your questions are important, no matter how small.").

□ Plan to include the family and significant others in the teaching session (when appropriate).

□ Plan for a quiet private environment that is conducive to learning.

□ Plan for active learning experiences (*i.e.*, use examples, simulations, games, and audiovisuals when appropriate).

□ Plan to pace learning. Don't give too much information at one time (*i.e.*, progress at the individual's learning pace).

□ Plan time to discuss progress (*e.g.*, ask the patient how he feels he is progressing and let him know how you feel he is progressing).

□ Plan time for summarizing what has been taught (*e.g.*, at the beginning of a session and at the end of a session).

Counseling as an Intervention

Counseling clients to help them make necessary changes or adjustments in their lives or to help them make choices about their health care is an important nursing activity. Counseling includes using teaching techniques to help the patient acquire the necessary knowledge to make decisions about his own health care. It also includes offering emotional and psychological support to the individual and his family as they seek to adjust to new circumstances of living. Through the use of teaching techniques and therapeutic communication, a nurse can offer her patient valuable psychological and intellectual support and can reduce the level of stress for both the patient and his family.

Consulting and Referring as an Intervention

Whenever the client's problems require more than independent nursing interventions, part of the nursing plan for interventions must be that of consulting with or referring to the appropriate health-care professional. For example, if the client states that he has trouble swallowing pills, a nurse might consult with the pharmacist to determine if there is a better method of giving the medications. If a person has a poor nutritional intake because he dislikes hospital food, the nurse should refer the problem to the hospital dietitian so that perhaps different meals can be served. Nurses must always refer medical problems and complications to physicians so that collaborative nursing interventions can be determined.

Determining Specific Interventions

Determining nursing interventions for specific nursing diagnoses involves determining the nursing actions or activities that will achieve the established expected outcomes. That is, what are you going to do to reduce or resolve each of the nursing diagnoses that you have identified?

There are three questions that are important to ask when determining nursing interventions for nursing diagnoses.

1. What is the cause (etiology) of the problem?
2. What can be done to eliminate or minimize the cause?
3. How can I help the client achieve the expected outcomes?

In order to determine nursing interventions for a potential or actual nursing diagnosis, you must identify its etiology and decide what can be done to reduce or eliminate it. How to identify the etiology of nursing diagnoses was discussed in Chapter 3 (see "Questions for Identifying the Etiology of a Health Problem). You should also remember from Chapter 3 that the etiology is found in the second clause of the problem statement for the nursing diagnosis (*i.e.*, after "related to"). Look at the example problem statement for *Fluid Volume Deficit related to insufficient fluid intake*.

Example Problem Statement

Fluid volume deficit related to \ insufficient fluid intake /
$\downarrow$
Second Clause (etiology)

Once you have determined the cause or contributing factors of the actual or potential nursing diagnosis, you must determine nursing interventions that would either eliminate the factors or minimize their effects. For example, if you identify the actual or potential diagnosis of *Impairment of Skin Integrity related to prescribed bed rest*, you should *determine interventions that would reduce the effect of the prescribed bed rest*. That is, you would plan a regimen of turning the patient from side to side and gently massaging areas that may receive more pressure than usual (*e.g.*, coccyx). If the diagnosis is described as a *potential* diagnosis, you would also have to establish a regimen of frequent focus assessments to be sure that the *potential* diagnosis has not become an *actual* diagnosis. If the diagnosis is described as an *actual* diagnosis, you should also plan to perform frequent focus assessments of the clinical manifestations of the diagnosis to monitor the status of the problem. For example, suppose you identified the actual nursing diagnosis of *Impairment of Skin Integrity related to prescribed bed rest as manifested by an area of red, scaly dry skin around the coccyx 2 inches in diameter*. You may plan to assess the area around the coccyx every 2 hours to assess for improvement or deterioration in the signs and symptoms.

If you identify a *possible* nursing diagnosis, then the interventions that you would prescribe would be those that would lead you to gain more information to help you to decide if the diagnosis is indeed present. For example, if you have identified the possible diagnosis of *Possible Ineffective Individual Coping*, you would prescribe interventions such as "Provide time for discussing how this individual feels that he is coping with his current problems."

Display 4-11 summarizes how to determine nursing interventions for actual, potential, and possible nursing diagnosis.

Display 4-11. *How to Determine Nursing Interventions for Actual, Potential, and Possible Nursing Diagnoses*

For an Actual Nursing Diagnosis:

1. Study the etiology (clause after "related to") and identify interventions that would reduce or remove the contributing factors.

2. Plan a regimen to perform frequent focus assessments of the clinical manifestations to monitor the status of the signs and symptoms of the problem.

Display 4-11. (Continued)

For a Potential Nursing Diagnosis:

1. Study the etiology and identify interventions that would reduce or remove the contributing factors.

2. Plan a regimen to perform frequent focus assessments to be sure that clinical manifestations have not appeared that would change the status of the diagnosis from potential to actual.

For a Possible Nursing Diagnosis:

1. Identify methods of collecting more data about the possible diagnosis to determine if any of the clinical manifestations or common contributing factors of the diagnosis are indeed present.

Considering Expected Outcomes to "Fine Tune" Nursing Interventions

In order to "fine tune" nursing interventions the expected outcomes of the plan of care should be considered as well as the etiology of the problem. For example, consider the example of *Fluid Volume Deficit related to insufficient fluid intake.* Studying the etiology should lead you to identify the nursing intervention of "increase fluid intake." Considering the expected outcome of "Will drink at least 2000 ml per day" will help you determine exactly how much fluid the person has to drink in order to prevent, reduce, or eliminate the problem. Considering both the etiology and the expected outcome will help you to determine exactly what nursing actions will help this particular patient achieve the expected outcomes.

☐ *Guidelines*

Planning Nursing Interventions/Actions

☐ Always perform a focus nursing assessment of the problem before determining appropriate nursing interventions.

☐ Look for interventions that will reduce or eliminate the etiology (cause) of the problem.

☐ Consider the expected outcome to be sure that your interventions are specific for that particular patient.

☐ Identify the strengths of the client and his family that can be encouraged so that they can participate in correcting the problem.

☐ Individualize nursing actions. What may work for one person may not for another.

☐ Be realistic. Nursing interventions should

Consider the patient's limitations/preferences

Consider the developmental age of the client

(continued)

☐ *Guidelines*

Be within the knowledge and capabilities of the nurse

Be congruent with other therapies

Provide safe and therapeutic environment

Utilize appropriate resources

☐ Utilize scientific rationale as a basis for your actions (*i.e., know why you are performing a nursing intervention*).

☐ Create opportunities for teaching and learning whenever possible (*e.g.,* teach the patient the reasons for the nursing actions that you have chosen).

☐ Consult other professionals when indicated (*e.g.,* dietitian).

☐ *Practice Session*

Determining Nursing Interventions for Nursing Diagnoses
(*suggested answers on page 168*)

For each of the nursing diagnoses and goals (outcome criteria) listed below, list some possible nursing interventions that would help the client to reach the set goal.

1. *Nursing Diagnosis:* Potential Impairment of Skin Integrity related to prescribed bed rest

   Outcome Criterion: Client will maintain good skin integrity while he is on bed rest.

   List appropriate nursing interventions:

2. *Nursing Diagnosis:* Potential for Ineffective Airway Clearance related to thoracic incision pain

   Outcome Criterion: Client will demonstrate effective coughing and deep breathing every 2 hours for the first day after surgery.

   List appropriate nursing interventions:

□ *Practice Session*

3. *Nursing Diagnosis:* Alteration in Bowel Elimination: Constipation related to insufficient exercise and inadequate fluid and roughage intake

   Outcome Criterion: Client will have daily soft bowel movements.

   List appropriate nursing interventions:

4. *Nursing Diagnosis:* Potential For Infection related to new incision

   Outcome Criteria: Incision will show no signs of infection (redness, swelling, drainage).

   Incision will be protected from microbial invasion by a clean, dry dressing at all times.

5. *Nursing Diagnosis:* Powerlessness related to hospitalization

   Outcome Criteria: Client will verbalize his feelings concerning being placed in the position of powerlessness while in the hospital.

   Client will be able to verbalize those things that he feels he should be allowed to control.

   Client will control his own care as much as possible.

(*continued*)

☐ *Practice Session*   6. In clinical conference (or with another nurse or student), choose a real patient, identify some nursing diagnoses and/or collaborative problems. List outcome criteria and some appropriate nursing interventions.

Determining Nursing Interventions for Collaborative Problems

According to Carpenito,* nursing interventions for collaborative problems are the following:

1. To perform frequent focus assessments to monitor the patient in order to detect possible or potential complications (*e.g.*, performing frequent neurological assessments of a client who has experienced a head injury to detect the possible complication of increased intracranial pressure)

2. To refer to physician when signs or symptoms of potential complications are present

3. To implement collaborative nursing interventions as prescribed by the physician (or other qualified health-care professional) (*e.g.*, irrigating a nasogastric tube every 2 hours with normal saline)

Monitoring to Detect Complications

Your ability to establish a regimen of performing focus assessments for monitoring to detect potential complications will depend on your nursing knowledge of disease process, medical and surgical treatments, diagnostic techniques, and monitoring modalities. For example, suppose you were caring for a patient who has just been admitted with severe burns and you identified the collaborative problem of *potential complication: hypovolemia.* You would have to know how to assess for hypovolemia (*i.e.*, take frequent vital signs, hourly urine output measurements, and read central venous pressures or Swan-Ganz catheter pressures). Often a physician will order how frequently an assessment should be recorded (*e.g.*, every hour). However, it is the nurse's responsibility to perform these assessments more frequently if she suspects an actual or impending complication, and to alert the physician about any changes in the patient's condition.

Monitoring to detect possible complications takes a high level of theoretical and technical knowledge. The following guidelines are suggested to help you determine exactly how you would monitor a given collaborative problem.

*Carpenito L: Personal communication, 1985

□ *Guidelines*   *Monitoring to Detect Potential Complications*

1. Always determine a base line (*i.e.,* determine what is the normal or current status of the problem in this specific situation).

   EXAMPLE:

   If you are monitoring the status of a patient on a respirator, consult with the physician or nurse specialist to determine the current acceptable arterial blood gases for this specific patient. What may be normal for this individual in this situation may be abnormal for another in a similar situation.

2. Determine how often focus assessments should be performed. This will depend on the status of the problem. Some institutions have standard acceptable regimens for monitoring specific problems.

   EXAMPLE:

   Many hospitals have standard routine orders for postoperative assessment of vital signs. However, if the problem seems to be unstable, it would be prudent to monitor it even more closely than the routine.

3. Determine early signs and symptoms of potential complications.

   EXAMPLE:

   Potential complication: hypovolemia. Early signs and symptoms would be increasing heart rate, drop in blood pressure, drop in urine output, and changes in mental status. You would assess for the presence of any of these signs and symptoms.

4. Determine exactly how and when focus assessments should be performed, and make sure all the nurses perform them in the same manner.

   EXAMPLE:

   All central venous pressure readings will be taken every hour with the patient flat in bed.

5. Determine the exact method of recording assessment findings for problem.

   EXAMPLE:

   Keeping a neurological assessment flow sheet that clearly describes neurological status

6. Determine what assessment findings would indicate possible deterioration in the patient's condition and would require you to notify the physician.

   EXAMPLE:

   Deciding that the physician should be notified if the patient has less than 30 ml of urine output for 2 consecutive hours

Implementing Nursing Interventions Prescribed by the Physician

Physicians' orders will often determine specific nursing interventions that will prevent potential complications. The following are some examples of specific nursing interventions that physicians frequently prescribe to prevent potential complications:

☐ Irrigating a nasogastric tube or Foley catheter to prevent it from becoming blocked by clots or sediment

☐ Maintaining suction for drainage tubes to facilitate drainage

☐ Administering anticoagulants to prevent thrombus formation

☐ Administering intravenous fluids to prevent dehydration or electrolyte imbalance

Before you implement nursing interventions ordered by a physician you should be sure that the order for the intervention is clear. In most cases, it should be clearly written, but there will be times when you, as a registered nurse, will be responsible for carrying out a verbal order. Whether the order is verbal or written, you should be sure to clarify the following:

☐ Exactly what intervention is to be done

☐ Exactly how the intervention is to be done

☐ Exactly when and how often it is to be done

☐ Exactly how much, how often, for how long, and by what route (in the case of medications or intravenous fluids)

☐ Exactly why the intervention is to be done. If you don't know why, then seek clarification through a review of the literature, consultation with an appropriate health-care professional, or by questioning the person who ordered the intervention.

The implementation of physicians' orders for specific nursing interventions is an important nursing role when caring for patients who are in an acute-care facility. In order to identify nursing diagnoses and collaborative problems for an individual who is hospitalized, you must be aware of the plan that the physician prescribes for your patient. You should routinely check for the presence of the following physicians' orders before you determine a plan of care:

☐ Diet/activity level

☐ Frequency of recording of vital signs, or other special assessment (*e.g.*, neuro checks)

☐ Medications/intravenous fluids

☐ Treatments/diagnostic studies

There are a few interventions that many physicians consider to be routine nursing interventions for some collaborative problems, and therefore may or may not be identified in the physician's orders. In some institutions, these become "unwritten rules," but they should be addressed in the standard care procedure manuals of the institution. Some examples of these interventions are listed below.

☐ Irrigating a nasogastric tube with saline every 2 hours

☐ Routine or special tracheostomy care

☐ Standard routine care of arterial and intravenous lines

You will have to become familiar with the standard care procedures at whatever facility you work because they will direct you in determining many of your collaborative interventions.

Using Standardized Care Plan Guides to Identify Client Outcomes and Nursing Interventions

Establishing goals and determining nursing interventions can be difficult for beginning nurses. However, today's nurses have an additional tool to help them in this complex task: the standardized care plan. As nurses have become more adept at researching and utilizing the nursing process, they have begun to generate standard care plans that can be used as a guide when identifying client outcomes and nursing interventions for certain situations. These standard care plans usually identify the common problems that are often seen with a given diagnosis. Standard care plans are now available from several different sources:

Institutional Care Plans. Many institutions maintain standard care plans on each unit. These care plans incorporate client outcomes and nursing interventions according to the unique standards of the institution.

Computerized Care Plans. These care plans can be broadly based on national standards but are often adapted specifically for a given institution.

Care Plans Printed in Books. Many books incorporate care plans that can be considered to be standard for a given medical or nursing diagnosis. Some are even written specifically with the intention of offering suggested standard care plans for nurses.*

---

*The following books are recommended for use as care plan guides:

Brunner LS, Suddarth DS: The Lippincott Manual of Nursing Practice, 4th ed. Philadelphia, JB Lippincott, 1986

Carpenito L: Nursing Diagnosis: Application to Clinical Practice. Philadelphia, JB Lippincott, 1983

Duke University Hospital Nursing Services: Duke Guidelines for Nursing Care: Process and Outcomes, 2nd ed. Philadelphia, JB Lippincott, 1983

All of the above can be valuable tools in helping you to establish a comprehensive, individualized plan of nursing care that clearly describes client outcomes and pertinent nursing interventions. However, you must be sure that you utilize these standard care plans as they are intended to be used. *They are to be used as a guide, not as a crutch.* When used correctly, suggested care plan guides can provide the nurse with some *basic* beginning information as she starts the care planning process. Using care plan guides helps to make the beginning work of care planning easier. Having this beginning work made easier helps to free the nurse to devote her time and creative energy to providing an individualized plan of care. You must carefully analyze the suggested care plan to determine what things are appropriate for your specific patient. Suggested standard care plans should always be used as a beginning, and never as an end. They should always be considered as beginning guides, never as set plans. Blindly using suggested care plans can be detrimental for your patient because it will be rare that all of your patient's specific problems will be addressed by one suggested care plan. Students and new graduates may find them to be valuable tools for learning, but they must be aware that *if they are used alone they can retard growth.* (Imagine if you only knew how to add, subtract, multiply, and divide by using a calculator!)

The following guidelines are suggested to help you to use standardized care plans for *individualized* client outcomes and in *individualized* nursing interventions.

☐ *Guidelines*   *Individualizing Standard Care Plans*

☐ Use only appropriate sources for your care plan guide. Ask yourself the following:

1. Is this standard care plan provided (or accepted) by the particular institution (or school) with which you are working? (Students and beginning nurses should check with their instructor or staff development nurse before using a standard care plan as a guide.)

2. Does the standard care plan source cite bibliographic information to validate its resources?

3. Is the standard care plan congruent with the standards of care set forth by the law, the ANA, and the institution where you are working?

☐ In order to reduce the temptation to use a standard care plan blindly, follow the steps below:

1. Always perform a complete nursing assessment and identify problems *yourself* first.

2. Once you have identified some problems yourself, check with the standard care plan to see if you have missed any of the problems that are associated with the ones that you have already diagnosed.

☐ *Guidelines*

3. Assess your patient for the presence of these problems.

4. List all the problems that you have identified, and establish expected outcomes (goals). You may want to compare your goals with the goals suggested by the standard care plan, but remember, goals must be highly specific and individualized.

5. Determine some nursing interventions *yourself* first.

6. Compare the interventions that you have identified with the interventions suggested by the standard care plan, and add any interventions that are appropriate for your patient. Delete interventions that are not appropriate.

Documenting the Plan of Nursing Care

Documenting the plan of nursing care, or writing the nursing care plan, is the final step in the planning process. If you fail to document your plan of nursing care, you waste all the effort that you have given to determining an individualized care plan for your patient. No one will know the work that has been done. Documenting the plan of care serves three purposes:

1. To validate that there has been a thorough plan of care formulated for each patient

2. To serve as a record that can later be studied to evaluate patient care

3. To communicate to other nurses the specific problems, goals, and interventions that have been identified for the patient

The importance of documenting the plan of care cannot be underestimated. Documentation is absolutely necessary for continuity of care and for later evaluation procedures. Most facilities today require that the documented care plan become a part of the client's permanent record so that it can be referred to when charting nursing notes or performing an evaluation. Good, clear documentation of the nursing care plan is the key to successful nursing audits. (Nursing audits consist of a complete formal evaluation of nursing care. Audits will be further addressed in Chapter 6, Evaluation.) Documenting the care plan includes listing the pertinent nursing diagnoses and collaborative problems, writing expected outcomes, writing nursing orders for nursing interventions, and recording periodic progress or evaluation reports.*

We have discussed how to correctly state nursing diagnoses, collaborative problems, and expected outcomes or goals. Let's look at the criteria for writing specific nursing orders.

---

* Recording periodic progress or evaluation reports will be discussed in Chapter 5, Implementation.

Writing Nursing Orders

Once you have determined the nursing interventions that you will employ in giving nursing care, you will need to write nursing orders so that all nurses caring for that particular patient will have clear instructions for implementing the plan of care. Because client teaching and client assessment should be employed as adjunct interventions to every nursing action, you should consider the following when writing nursing orders:

☐ What to look for (assessment)

☐ What to do

☐ What to teach

For example, suppose you were caring for a patient who had a hernia repair, and you had identified *Potential Ineffective Airway Clearance related to smoking.* You probably would plan to assist him with breathing and coughing exercises for the first few days after surgery. To write the order for this intervention, you should consider what you want the nurses to look for (assessment), what you want them to do, and what you want them to teach. For this situation, the order may look like this:

1. Assess for rales/rhonchi/increased mucus production every 4 hours.
2. Assist the person to perform coughing and breathing exercises with pillow and hand over incision for support every 4 hours.
3. Reinforce (teach) the person the importance of coughing and deep breathing.

Nursing orders may not always need to describe assessment and teaching as well as the activity to be performed, but if you routinely consider *assessing, doing,* and *teaching* you are more likely to write comprehensive nursing orders that encompass more than just the activity that is to be performed.

"Fine Tuning" Nursing Orders.   Nursing orders must be specific and clear. They should include the following:

☐ Date: The date the order was written

☐ Verb: Action to be performed

☐ Subject: Who is to do it

☐ Descriptive phrase: How, when, where, how often, how long, how much

☐ Signature: Whoever wrote the order should sign it.

EXAMPLE:

☐ Date: 1/2/86

☐ Verb: assist

☐ Who: Mr. Jones

☐ Descriptive phrase: To sit on the side of the bed three times a day for 10 minutes

☐ Signature: H. Laird, RN

This order would look like this on the nursing care plan:

1/26/86   Assist Mr. Jones* to sit on the side of the bed for 10 minutes t.i.d.

M. Riley RN

If you added the dimensions of assessing and teaching to this order, the orders may look like this:

1/26/86   Assist to sit on the side of the bed three times a day for 10 minutes.

—Assess for dizziness or fatigue

—Teach the importance of gradual increase in activity level.   M. Riley RN

Display 4-12 shows how you would write specific nursing orders for a given nursing action.

Display 4-12. *Nursing Actions with Corresponding Nursing Orders*

Nursing Action	Nursing Orders
Ambulate patient.	Ambulate patient the length of the hall using the walker three times a day.
Maintain caloric intake of 3,000 calories/day.	Consult dietitian to plan meals and snacks.
	Encourage patient to complete all his meals.
	Offer between-meal milkshakes (likes chocolate and strawberry) t.i.d.
	Have the patient keep a daily record of food eaten.
Provide for periods of uninterrupted rest.	Do not awaken from 12 MN to 7 AM—allow to rest from 1 PM to 3 PM (no visitors).

*The patient's name may be omitted because it is understood who the patient is (*e.g.*, "Assist to sit. . .")

□ *Practice Session*   *Writing Nursing Orders*
                          (suggested answers on page 170)

For each nursing intervention listed below, write appropriate nursing orders.

1. Maintain a program of turning from side to side.

2. Force fluids to 3000 ml a day.

3. Encourage patient to express her feelings.

4. Encourage daily bowel elimination.

☐ *Practice Session*   5. Get patient out of bed daily b.i.d.

Forms for Documenting Nursing Care Plans

Forms and methods of documenting care plans vary from institution to institution because they must be tailor-made to meet the needs of the nurses and clients in each unique setting. You will have to familiarize yourself with the method used by the institution in which you'll be working. However, there are certain common components that should be present in order to direct nursing care. Each nursing care plan should have the following components:

☐ Nursing diagnoses/collaborative problems

☐ Long-term discharge goals (client outcomes)

☐ Short-term client goals (outcomes)

☐ Nursing orders (interventions)

☐ Evaluation (progress reports)

Many hospitals use a nursing Kardex for documentation of the plan of care. A Kardex is a type of metal flip chart that contains all the care plans for all of the patients on a given unit. The Kardex care plan form itself is usually made of white cardboard and is about 8 inches × 11 inches, which is then folded in half. Although a few hospitals still use pencil for their Kardex care plans, it is recommended that they be written in ink so they can become a permanent part of the patient's chart.

Some hospitals no longer keep the care plans on a nursing Kardex. In these agencies, the care plans are usually kept either on a clip board at the patient's bedside or on the patient's chart.

The following show several sample care plans. One is organized according to the specific needs of a given hospital. The others are organized according to Orem's theory of self-care and Gordon's functional health patterns. Note that all of the necessary components of the nursing care plan are present (nursing diagnoses/collaborative problems, expected outcomes, nursing orders, and progress or evaluation summaries).

(Text continues on page 129)

Sample Care Plan Organized According to Orem's Self-Care Theory
Health Focus: Life Cycle
Long-Term Goal: Mrs. J. will react with other residents and become more involved in activities by 12/5/85.

Assessment Data	Nursing Diagnosis/ Collaborative Problem
10/15/85 *Therapeutic self-care demand:* Universal/Balance between activity & rest. *Related signs and symptoms:* Sleeps in a chair much of the day. States she's bored. Affect is flat. *Strengths:* Alert, oriented, pleasant, clear. Communicates well. Enjoys company, TV, gardening, music. Knowledgeable. *Limitations:* Has chronic low back pain. Confined to wheel chair. *Self-care deficit (knowledge, attitude, skills):* Lack of environmental stimuli and activity	Diversional Activity Deficit R/T inability to perform ADL as manifested by statements of "there's nothing I can do here."
10/15/85 *Therapeutic self-care demand:* Health deviation: back pain. *Related signs and symptoms:* c/o constant low back pain & asking for "pain killers." States she wishes she could control pain. *Strengths:* Willing to learn & do anything to reduce pain so she can walk independently again. Aware of effects of immobility. *Limitations:* Anxious, advanced age, Hx of partial compression fx L1, prosthesis r. hip, little family support. *Self-care deficit: (knowledge, attitude, skills):* Lacks knowledge of pain management techniques.	Impaired Physical Mobility R/T pain

(Adapted from Holy Family College Nursing Department, Philadelphia, PA)

Outcome	Nursing System/ Nursing Orders	Progress/Evaluation
10/15/85 1. Will report activities she enjoys doing by 10/16/85. 2. Will perform at least 2 activities a day by 10/20/85. 3. Will report less boredom by 10/20. 4. Will sleep 8 hrs. at night by 10/20.	Nursing System: Partially compensatory Nursing Orders: 10/15/85 1. Assess activity level. 2. Suggest some activities to do (likes playing Bingo, cards, & watching out window). 3. Encourage her to make suggestions and express ideas. 4. Maintain lighted, cheerful environment. 5. Make daily routine as normal as possible. M. Malloon, RN	States she likes Bingo, cards, synagog, sitting by window. MM 10/20/85 Will attend Bingo and goes to synagog if encouraged. MM Attended exercise class, but needs constant encouragement. MM States she enjoys the activities, but she does not seem to remember much about them. Sleeping 6–8 hours most nights. MM
1. Will report lessening of pain using a five point scale by 10/25. 2. Will discuss techniques for ↓ pain experience by 10/25. 3. Will be less dependent on medications by 10/25. 4. Will verbalize importance of ambulating by 10/18. 5. Will attempt to take small steps with walker by 10/25.	Nursing System: Partially compensatory Nursing Orders: 10/15/85 1. Assess low back pain q shift and report abnormalities (e.g., edema, bruising, redness). 2. Massage q 4 hrs. 3. Perform ROM. 4. Encourage her to wear brace OOB. 5. Medicate prn. Coach her in relaxation techniques. 6. Assist her to walk with walker t.i.d. M. Malloon, RN	10/25 Rates pain at #2 level (less). MM Relates that back rubs & massages reduce pain. MM Still needs medication q 4 hr. MM 10/18 Verbalizes that she should try to walk more to keep up strength. MM 10/25 Can walk from bed to bathroom with walker. MM

**Sample Care Plan Organized According to Gordon's Functional
Health Patterns**

Assessment Data	Nursing Diagnosis/ Collaborative Problem
10/20/85 *Health management/Health perception:* Nonsmoker. Goes to aerobic 3 × wk when well. States being ill and dependent on others is very difficult on her.	10/20/85 1. Fluid volume deficit R/T Fever, diarrhea, and loss of appetite as manifested by dark concentrated urine.
Nutrition/metabolic pattern: 20£ overweight. Has had no appetite since illness started 10 days ago. Has had fever of 101 much of the time. Skin intact—no rashes.	
Elimination pattern: BM q other day usually. Now has diarrhea × 10–15 per day. Has external hemorrhoids. Urine dark and concentrated.	2. Alteration in bowel elimination R/T unknown etiology.
Activity/exercise pattern: Has not been out of house for past 10 days. Feels she is too weak to go out.	
Cognitive perception pattern: College graduate. Alert and appropriate in communication.	
10/20/85 *Sleep/rest pattern:* Sleeps much of the time, but disturbed by having to get up to BR for diarrhea	10/20/85 3. Possible alteration in family processes R/T illness of mother 4. Potential impairment of skin integrity (rectal area) R/T diarrhea & hemorrhoids.
Self-perception/self-concept pattern: States she's an independent individual.	
Role/relationship pattern: Married. Has one child. Worried because she says husband is "not good" with daughter.	
Sexual/reproductive pattern: Married. Other data collection deferred.	
Coping/stress pattern: States she's a "doer"—likes to be active doing things when she is depressed.	
Value/belief pattern: Catholic. Attends Mass most Sundays.	

Outcome	Nursing Orders	Evaluation
Will maintain hydration by drinking at least 2000 ml per day every day.	10/20/85 1. Keep ginger ale with juice at bedside. 2. Force fluids (clear liq) to: 1000 ml (7–3) 750 ml (3–11) 250 ml (7–11) 3. Assess fluid intake every 2 hours while awake. 4. Both nurse & pt should keep a record of I/O. 5. Monitor electrolyte studies. J. Martin RN	10/22 Fluid intake only 1500 ml last 2 days. Discussed her need to push more. JM Electrolytes WNL JM Urine output 700cc and concentrated. JM Keeping own I/O record. JM
Will develop normal bowel movements by controlling diarrhea through medication and diet by 10/22.	10/20/85 1. Maintain clear liquid diet. 2. Assess BMs q 3° while awake and give Lomotil prn. J. Martin RN	10/22 Diarrhea ↓ to 4 × day. Clear liquids maintained. Taking Lomotil q.i.d. JM
She and her husband will discuss how family will cope with illness by 10/22.	10/20/85 Spend time discussing with husband and wife together and separately to determine how the family is adapting to illness and to identify potential problems. J. Martin RN	10/22 Husband has not been to visit for longer than 10 minutes, and I have missed him both times. Told her to ask him to call me when he can. JM
Rectal area will remain clean and without signs of irritation.	Encourage warm sitz baths qid especially p̄ BMs J. Martin RN	10/22 Taking sitz bath. Rectal area clean—not red. JM

Sample Care Plan Organized by the Need of the Individual Institution

Date of Admission: 8/24 **Reason for Admission:** Was involved in 2 car accident (no one else injured) and suffered ® rib fracture c̄ hemo-pneumothorax

Discharge Goal: To return to home to recuperate; to be able to do own ADL.

Age: 29 **Occupation:** Construction worker **Household Members:** Wife & baby girl **Religion:** Prot.

Nursing Diagnosis/ Problem	Client Outcome (Goal)	Target Date	Nursing Orders	Evaluation/ Progress
8/24 1. Potential Fluid Volume Deficit related to poor fluid intake as manifested by verbalizing that he hates to drink H_2O	Will drink at least 2000 ml daily	q shift	8/25/85 1. Encourage fluid intake to 2000 ml/ day as follows: 8^A-4^P = 1000 ml 4^P-12^A = 700 ml 12^A-8^A = 300 ml 2. Offer OJ, cranberry juice, iced tea (dislikes H_2O & milk). 3. Keep 7-Up at bedside. 4. Have him keep a record of daily fluid intake. B. MacIntyre RN	8/25 Needs much encouragement, but does drink. BM 8/25 Keeping written record. BM
8/25 2. Potential Ineffective Airway Clearance related to pain from incisional site as manifested by a weak cough effort and statements of pain c̄ cough	Will cough and deep breathe q 2° for 2 days	q shift	8/25/85 1. Offer pain med ½° before coughing session. 2. Splint incision c̄ pillow. 3. Reinforce importance of coughing. 4. Assist c̄ coughing q 2°. B. MacIntyre RN	8/25 Cough is still weak. Needs much encouragement. Productive of thick white mucus. BM 8/26 Improved cough effort. Cough productive as above. BM
8/26 3. Immobility related to bed rest and chest tubes as manifested by restrictive chest tubes.	Will turn and reposition himself q 2°	q shift	8/26/85 1. Assist to reposition himself q 2°—has trouble lying on ® side. 2. Reinforce the importance of moving while in bed. 3. Encourage movement of legs q 2° B. MacIntyre RN	8/26 Moves well c̄ assistance BM

☐ *Guidelines*   *Documenting Care Plans*

☐ Be sure that diagnoses, expected outcomes, nursing orders, and evaluation are addressed on each care plan.

☐ List only those nursing diagnoses and collaborative problems that vary from routine or standard care.

☐ Be brief, but be clear:

Use accepted abreviations (*e.g.*, NPO, OOB).

Use key words rather than full sentences.

Refer nurses to procedure manuals for routine and standard care procedures.

☐ List long- and short-term goals (when appropriate), and set target dates for goal achievement.

☐ Indicate dates when goals are set and met.

Problem-Oriented Medical Records (POMR)

Some institutions use *Problem-Oriented Medical Records* (POMR) to document the plan of care. POMR is a method of charting the patient's plan of care whereby all members of the health-care team document patient problems in the same place on the chart (called the problem list). For example, if you were to look at the problem list for a particular patient, you may find problems that have been identified by physicians, nurses, dietitians, and physical therapists. The problems are listed in order of when they were identified, not necessarily in order of priority. Display 4-13 shows a sample problem list.

Display 4-13.   *Problem List*

Date of Diagnosis	Problem	Date Resolved
1/5/86	1. Cerebrovascular accident (identified by physician)	
	2. Potential Impairment of Skin Integrity related to immobility (identified by nursing)	
	3. Unsteady gait (identified by physical therapist)	

(continued)

Display 4-13. *(Continued)*

1/7/86	4. Alteration in Self-Concept related to loss of ability to move right side (identified by nursing)	
1/8/86	5. Urinary tract infection (identified by physician)	1/13/86

Institutions that use POMR feel that listing all the problems in one place will increase communication among the members of the health-care team; each member working with the patient will be aware of *all* of the problems for that particular patient.

SOAP Charting

The use of POMR requires that all members of the health-care team use a method of charting called SOAP charting. SOAP charting includes documentation of the following information on the patient's chart:

S = Subjective data (what the patient tells you about his problem)

O = Objective data (what is observed about the patient's problem)

A = Assessment/analysis (problem statement)

P = Plan (goals and interventions)

Display 4-14 shows an example of SOAP charting.

Display 4-14. *SOAP Charting*

S: "I feel so helpless because I can't move since I had my stroke."

O: Unable to move right side of body
   Slouched in bed in half sitting position
   Has reddened area about 5 cm around coccyx

A: Potential Impairment of Skin Integrity related to immobility

P: Prevent skin breakdown:

   Reposition side to side every 2 hours when in bed.

   Assist out of bed three times a day for ½ hour.

   Acquire sheepskin for coccyx area.

   Massage coccyx with lotion q.i.d. and p.r.n.

SOAPIE Charting

SOAPIE charting, an expanded form of SOAP charting, is closer to the nursing process in format because it includes the steps of implementation and evaluation.

S = Subjective data

O = Objective data

A = Assessment

P = Plan

I = Implementation (interventions)

E = Evaluation

At present, SOAP charting is often used for the initial assessment of the patient, and SOAPIE charting is used after implementation of the care has progressed to the point at which evaluation is appropriate.

□ *Key Points*

Planning Nursing Care

1. The third step of the nursing process, planning, involves the following activities:

    Setting priorities (See Display 4-1 and Guidelines: Setting Priorities.)

    Establishing client goals/expected outcomes (See Display 4-6 and Display 4-8 and Guidelines: Establishing Goals/Outcomes.)

    Determining nursing actions (See Guidelines: Planning Nursing Interventions/Actions.)

    Documenting the nursing care plan (See Guidelines: Documenting Care Plans.)

2. When you establish a plan of nursing care, you must apply standards that are set by the law, the ANA, and the institution where you are working.

3. Establishing goals (expected outcomes) is a necessary part of the planning phase for two reasons:

    Both the client and the health-care team need to know what must be accomplished in order to resolve or reduce the diagnosed problems.

    The established goal or outcome can later be studied to evaluate how well the plan of care is working (*i.e.*, is the goal being met?).

4. A specific client outcome must be written for each nursing diagnosis or collaborative problem that has been identified.

5. Writing expected outcomes involves writing goals in three domains:

    Cognitive domain: Outcomes that are associated with changes in knowledge or intellectual abilities

    Affective domain: Outcomes that are associated with changes in attitudes, feelings, or values

    Psychomotor domain: Outcomes that deal with developing motor skills

    Verbs used in writing expected outcomes/goals should be measurable verbs that describe the exact behavior that you expect to *see* or *hear*.

(continued)

☐ *Key Points*

6. Planning nursing actions includes planning interventions that prevent complications and that promote, maintain, and restore health.

7. Nursing interventions include assessing, doing, and teaching. (See Guidelines: Planning Patient Teaching.)

8. Nursing orders should give clear instructions about what nursing actions should be implemented for each specific problem, including the following components:

    Date: The date the order was written

    Verb: The action that is to be performed

    Subject: Who is going to perform the action

    Descriptive phrase: How, when, where, how often, how long, how much

    Signature of the nurse: Whoever wrote it should sign it.

9. Standard care plans should be used only *as a guide* with thoughtful analysis on your part as a nurse. (See Guidelines: Individualizing Standard Care Plans.)

10. Methods of documenting care plans vary from institution to institution because they must meet the unique needs of the nurses and patients. However, they should all provide for documentation of nursing diagnoses/collaborative problems, expected outcomes, nursing interventions, and evaluation.

11. Documentation of the nursing care plan is essential for continuity of nursing care and for any type of evaluation procedure.

☐ *Bibliography*

American Nurses' Association: Standards of Nursing Practice. Kansas City, MO, American Nurses' Association, 1973

Carpenito L: Nursing Diagnosis: Application to Clinical Practice. Philadelphia, JB Lippincott, 1983

Gordon M: Nursing Diagnosis: Process and Application. New York, McGraw-Hill, 1982

Griffith J, Christensen P: Nursing Process: Application of Theories, Frameworks and Models. St Louis, CV Mosby, 1982

Kozier B, Erb G: Fundamentals of Nursing: Concepts and Process. Menlo Park, CA, Addison-Wesley, 1979

Maslow A: Motivation in Personality. New York, Harper & Row, 1970

Orem, D: Nursing: Concepts of Practice, 2nd ed. New York, McGraw-Hill, 1980

Popkess S: Diagnosing your patient's strengths. Nursing '81 11:34–37, 1981

Potter P, Perry A: Fundamentals of Nursing Concepts: Concepts, Process, and Practice. St Louis, CV Mosby, 1985

Van Hoozer H, Ruther L, Craft M: Introduction to Charting. Philadelphia, JB Lippincott, 1982

☑ Continuing data collection
☑ Performing nursing interventions
☑ Documenting nursing care (charting)
☑ Giving verbal nursing reports
☑ Maintaining a current care plan

5

Implementation

Standard V: *Nursing actions provide for client/patient participation in health promotion, maintenance, and restoration.*

Standard VI: *Nursing actions assist the client/patient to maximize his health capabilities.* *

*Abstracted from Standards—Nursing Practice. Copyright American Nurses' Association, 1973

□ *Glossary*   ***Charting***   The concise, accurate, factual, written documentation and communication of occurrences and situations pertaining to a particular client (Van Hoozer et al., 1982)

Implementation   The process of putting a plan into action

The fourth step of the nursing process is *implementation*. It is during this phase that you will actually carry out the plan that has been set forth. In other words, you will be putting the plan into action. Implementation involves the following activities:

□ Continuing data collection and assessment
□ Performing nursing interventions
□ Documenting nursing care (charting)
□ Giving verbal nursing reports
□ Maintaining a current care plan

Relationship of Planning to Implementation

Planning and implementation are often so closely related that you may find that when you are in the clinical setting the planning stage of the nursing process may seem to have been omitted, with nursing actions being performed immediately after assessment and diagnosis. For example, if a nurse identifies an urgent problem such as respiratory difficulty, she may begin nursing interventions immediately after she has identified the problem (*e.g.*, raising the head of the bed and repositioning the patient). Planning may seem to have been omitted, but in actuality the nurse is making a quick mental plan as she implements nursing actions.

Continuing Data Collection and Assessment

When you implement nursing actions, it is important to remember that *you must continue to collect pertinent data and assess the behaviors of your patient while you are giving nursing care*. The time that you spend performing specific or routine nursing activities can be a valuable time for further data collection. For example, the simple procedure of giving a bed bath or back rub can yield important data about the physical and mental status of your patient. During these procedures, you can gain information about your patient's physical status by making observations such as the condition of his skin and his ability to move; and you can gain information about his mental status by using therapeutic communication techniques to encourage him to verbalize feelings or concerns. Note the following example:

During the nursing report, the evening nurse had been told that Mrs. Sowers seemed to be a somewhat "difficult" patient. She had been admitted for studies of her gastrointestinal tract, but was otherwise in good general health. Mrs. Sowers spent the entire day in bed, and the nursing staff had been concerned because they had decided that she should be ambulating to maintain her strength. However, Mrs. Sowers had verbalized that she was too tired to walk much and that she wanted to rest in bed. The nurses had described her as being a somewhat dependent person who was very quiet and introverted. That evening, the nurse went in to give Mrs. Sowers a back rub and to help her get settled for bed. While giving the back rub, the nurse mentioned to Mrs. Sowers that she seemed very tired all the time. She then asked if there was something that was causing her to feel this way. Mrs. Sowers responded by explaining that she had not slept well in weeks because she had just found out her daughter had breast cancer and she was very frightened that she might die. This was important information that had never been offered before. The nurse was then able to talk with Mrs. Sowers about her fears and concerns and to offer a positive outlook by explaining that breast cancer, when detected early, has a good prognosis. By ten o'clock that night, Mrs. Sowers was not only up ambulating, but also helping her roommate by offering her sips of juice, and so forth.

The above situation exemplifies the importance of ongoing data collection during implementation of nursing actions.

Performing Nursing Interventions

Nursing interventions are those activities performed by the nurse and the client to prevent illness (or its complications) and to promote, maintain, or restore health. Performing nursing interventions includes the following:

☐ Directly performing an activity for a client

☐ Assisting the client to perform an activity himself

☐ Supervising the client (or family) while he performs an activity himself

☐ Teaching the client (or family) about his health care

☐ Counseling the client (or family) in making choices about seeking and utilizing appropriate health-care resources

☐ Monitoring (assessing) the client for potential complications of illness

Chapter 4 (Planning) discusses how to determine specific nursing interventions for specific problems. This section will discuss how interventions, in general, should be implemented.

The tasks involved in performing nursing interventions can vary from simple to complex. However, there are some activities that are common to almost all interventions. The nonsensical word "cwipat" is suggested to help you to remember the common tasks that you should perform with every nursing intervention. "Cwipat" stands for the following:

C = *C*heck the orders and equipment.

W = *W*ash your hands.

I = *I*dentify the patient.

P = *P*rovide for safety and privacy.

A = *A*ssess the problem.

T = *T*ell the person or *T*each the person about what you are going to do.

Making sure that you do all the steps suggested by the word "cwipat" before you perform a nursing intervention helps to organize the nursing procedure and reduce the possibility of error.

The following guidelines are suggested to help you when implementing (performing) nursing interventions.

☐ *Guidelines*   *Implementing (Performing) Nursing Interventions*

☐ Never perform a nursing intervention until you know the reason (rationale) for performing the activity, the expected effect of the activity, the possible side-effects of the activity, and the possible adverse effects of the activity.

☐ Before you implement a nursing action, you must reassess your patient to determine the status of the problem and whether the interventions previously identified are still valid (*i.e.*, perform a focus assessment).

☐ Performing nursing interventions cannot be a rote or mechanical activity—you must continually assess the response of the patient to your nursing interventions and be ready to change interventions that are not working.

☐ When you perform nursing interventions, you should include the patient and his family—always explain why you are performing the intervention.

☐ Nursing interventions should be accomplished in a safe and therapeutic environment. Plan ahead to be sure the environment is appropriate for whatever activity is going to be performed.

☐ When implementing nursing interventions, be sure that you are aware of institutional protocols and procedures, which often vary from institution to institution.

Documenting Nursing Care (Charting)

Charting, or documentation of nursing care, is a legal requirement of all health-care systems. There are no ifs, ands or buts—you must learn to chart, and you must learn to chart well. The nurses' notes that you will be writing will become a part of the client's permanent legal record, a record that may later be introduced as evidence in a court of law. These notes will be the most current written communication of what has happened to the patient during the course of a given day. Poor, illegible, or incomplete charting may impede nursing care because it will be more difficult to recognize significant changes in health status without the clear documentation of client activities and behaviors. Good, factually descriptive nursing notes will enhance patient care because they will communicate the pertinent aspects of the client's health care and help others to assess patterns of client responses.

You will notice that forms used for charting nurses' notes will vary because each health-care facility needs to have a method of documentation that meets its particular requirements. Even though these forms may differ in appearance, they must all provide for documentation of observations and occurrences according to exact time and sequence of events—often this documentation will provide the only answers to questions that may arise about a client's health care. Nurses' notes may offer the only proof that medical and nursing treatments have indeed been carried out. This information may later be necessary for insurance purposes and for evaluation of nursing care.

Just as with nursing assessments, there are two types of nurses' notes. One is the comprehensive nurses' notes that are written at the time of the initial contact with a given client, and the other is the problem-focused nurses' notes that are written concerning specific problems. See the accompanying examples of comprehensive admission nursing notes and problem-focused nursing notes that have been written for a patient who has the nursing diagnosis of *Potential Ineffective Airway Clearance related to thick secretions* (page 138).

You will notice a big difference in the amount of information that is charted with each type of nurses' notes. Patients with more acute and complex problems will require more frequent, in-depth, and comprehensive nursing notes. Patients with less severe problems are more likely to require problem-focused nursing notes that are shorter and less comprehensive.

As you move from one health-care facility to another, you will have to become familiar with both the charting forms and the responsibilities for charting that are set forth by the policies and procedures of each particular setting. Although the forms, policies, and procedures may differ from place to place, the basic content of nurses' notes is quite similar. The guidelines on page 139 are suggested to help you to learn how to write good nurses' notes in any facility.

Example of Comprehensive Admission Nurses' Notes

Date and Time	Of Special Notation	Nursing Assessments and Comments
6/86 7:30PM	$98^5-\dfrac{\text{irreg}}{120}-32$ No known allergies Note medications ⟶	Admission Note: _____ Admitted this 71 y.o. female from the e.r. via stretcher $\bar{c}$ a diagnosis of CHF + atrial fib. Ht 5'1" Wt. 121# _____ BP Ⓛ arm $120/_{84}$ BP Ⓡ arm $118/_{84}$ _____ States she takes digoxin 0.25 mg OD. _____ Last taken this a.m. @ 10AM. Takes no other meds. _____
7:35	Resp: Card: Circ: GI: GU: Skeletal: Skin: Mental Status:	Lungs $\bar{c}$ scattered rales bilat. O_2 on @3 l/min via cannula. Denies history of smoking. Coughing up frothy white mucus. _____ Monitor shows atrial fib at 120 $\bar{c}$ occasional PVCs. No murmur or rub. Denies chest pain. Skin wm and moist. Peripheral pulses satisfactory. Heparin lock intact Ⓡarm. _____ Bowel sounds ⊕—denies discomfort. _____ Foley catheter draining clear yellow urine. _____ States she has arthritis in both shoulders. Clear, no rashes or pressure points noted. Alert, oriented. Stated that she was relieved to be in the hospital where they could "watch my heart." _____
8PM	$-\dfrac{\text{irreg}}{124}-32$ Lasix 40 mg IV	See care plan for nursing diagnosis. H. Laird RN Resting—monitor, respiration unchanged.
9PM	$98^4-\dfrac{\text{irreg}}{100}-28$ Dr. O'Hara vs & exam	Foley⟶diuresing well. Respirations— improved. _____ H. Laird RN

Example of Problem-Focused Nurses' Notes

Date and Time	Problems/Diagnoses	Nursing Assessments and Comments
6/86 8AM	#1 Potential Ineffective Airway Clearance related to thick secretions #2 Potential for fluid volume deficit related to poor fluid intake	Coughing up thick white mucus—he does this well, but needs to be reminded to work at it. Lungs have a few scattered rhonchi. Fluids encouraged—he does drink juices well—apple juice on ice kept at bedside. - H. Laird RN
10:30AM		OOB to chair for ½ hour. States he feels very fatigued, but he is steady on his feet.
10:45AM	VD-550ml	Voided lge amount clear yellow urine. Allowed to rest before pulmonary function test. _____ H. Laird RN
11:30AM		To special studies via wheelchair for pulmonary function. _____ H. Laird RN
12:30PM		Returned via wheelchair. Assisted back to bed. Ate all of his lunch—said it was the first time he's been hungry. _____ H. Laird RN

☐ *Guidelines*   *Charting Nurses' Notes*

☐ Use ink and be legible. Print if your handwriting is not clear.

☐ Write your notes as soon as possible after giving nursing care so that your recall will be most accurate.

☐ Be precise. Write down exactly how, when, and where the events and activities occurred.

EXAMPLE:

"7/11/86, 9:10 P.M.—Admitted to room 321A from the E.R. via stretcher accompanied by wife and Dr. Willens."

☐ Always sign your first initial, last name, and credentials after each entry that you complete (*e.g.*, F. Nightingale, R.N.).

☐ Never leave a blank line—draw a line through unused spaces before your signature. (Note the example below.)

Date Time	Vital Signs			B/P	Fluids		Nursing Notes
	Temp	Pulse	Resp.		Intake	Output	
4/20/86	98⁴	92	20		78	200	Assisted to B.R. Refused bkfst. c/o
7:30AM							nausea. S. Jones R.N.———
8:30AM		88	20				A.M. care given Abd. dsg. dry.
							S. Jones R.N.———
9:45AM		84	16				Dr. Witt here. S. Jones R.N.———
10:50AM	98⁴	110	20				c/o shooting, sharp incisional pain.
							Quarter size pink drainage noted on
							abd. dsg. Requests pain med.———
							S. Jones R.N.———

☐ Include the following in your nurses' notes:

Assessment: What you see, hear, smell, or observe about the current physical and emotional status of the client

Intervention: The activities performed by the client, yourself, family, or other members of the health-care team

Evaluation: The response of the client to activities and interventions performed

☐ Be concise, yet descriptive. You don't have to write complete sentences, but use adjectives and accepted abbreviations to give a good picture of activities and observations.

(*continued*)

☐ *Guidelines*

EXAMPLE:

Wrong: Ambulated about room

Right: Needs encouragement, but ambulated well with assistance about room

☐ Be specific. Avoid using vague terms.

EXAMPLE:

Wrong: Noted moderate amount of drainage on abdominal dressing

Right: Abdominal dressing has an area of light pink drainage about 6 inches in diameter.

☐ Be complete—remember the adage, "if it wasn't charted, it wasn't done." If you fail to chart medications or other actions delivered *or* withheld, it may result in an adverse reaction, overdose, or perhaps even death.

☐ Use examples and the client's own words to clarify your description of what you observe or infer.

EXAMPLE:

Wrong: "Appears uncomfortable"

Right: "Doesn't seem to get good pain relief—he states that he is 'OK' but he moves stiffly and constantly holds his side."

☐ Always document variations from the norm (*e.g.*, abnormalities in respiration, circulation, mental status or behavior).

☐ Always document the status of invasive lines/treatment modalities (*e.g.*, oxygen therapy, traction, Foley catheters, nasogastric tubes, intravenous lines).

☐ Don't use the word "patient." Since it's the patient's chart, it is assumed.

☐ *Practice Session*

Charting Nurses' Notes
(suggested answers on page 171)

Study the two case situations listed below. Then, using the form provided on pages 142–143 (or using your own form), write the nursing notes that you would record, given the data presented for each situation.

Case I

Today you are Mr. Johns' nurse. He is a smoker and was admitted 2 days ago with chronic lung disease. He has the nursing diagnosis of Potential Ineffective Airway Clearance related to thick mucus secretions. When you enter his room at 8:30 A.M., he is sitting in a chair and seems to be wheezing more than usual. You note that he is using accessory muscles of the chest to help him breathe. His breakfast tray is sitting in front of him untouched. When you tell him that he seems to be having more trouble breathing, he replies, "Nope, I'm okay—I'm just a little tired, that's all." He refuses to eat because he says he's not hungry.

Ten minutes later, you enter the room to take his vital signs. His temperature is 97°F. His pulse is 130 and regular. His blood pressure is 170/94. His respiratory status is essentially unchanged with a rate of 32, but his behavior has changed. He is now more restless and is not sure that he is still in the hospital. You assist him into bed, put up the side rails, raise the head of the bed, and begin oxygen at 2 liters/min via nasal cannula. He still appears to be in respiratory distress. You notify the physician about these changes.

At 9:00 A.M., the physician examines the patient and orders arterial blood gases to be drawn by the lab and breathing treatments to begin immediately.

At 9:10 A.M., the lab draws blood gases and asks you to maintain pressure on the arterial puncture site for 5 minutes. You do this, and note that the site has no bleeding after 5 minutes.

At 9:15 A.M., the respiratory therapist comes in and administers the breathing treatment. Mr. Johns then coughs up a large amount of thick white mucus.

At 9:35 A.M., you reassess Mr. Johns and find that his lungs are more clear. He no longer seems confused, and he agrees to take a few sips of water.

At 10:00 A.M., Mr. Johns is much improved and asks to get out of bed. You discontinue his oxygen and assist him to a chair. His pulse is 110, and respirations are 28.

Case II

Tonight you are Mrs. Fox's nurse. Mrs. Fox is a newly diagnosed diabetic who has the nursing diagnosis of Knowledge Deficit: Self-administration of insulin.

You have taught Mrs. Fox how to give her own insulin injection, and she has given herself her first injection that morning without problems. You walk into the room at 5:00 P.M. to supervise her in giving herself her pre-dinner insulin. Mrs. Fox follows the procedure for withdrawing the insulin, but contaminates the needle before she injects herself. You point this out to her, and she replies, "Well, it only barely touched the sheet when I put it down for a moment." You reinforce the importance of maintaining sterile technique.

She eats all of her dinner. At 8:00 P.M., she states that she's "dying for a chocolate bar" and that she feels that the diabetic diet is going to be impossible to follow. You discuss the possibility of talking with the dietitian concerning possible modifications in diet and point out that she is scheduled for a fruit snack at 9:00 P.M. You suggest that perhaps she could do something to get her mind off her desire for food. She decides to call her friend on the phone to chat.

(Practice Session continues on page 144)

Date and Time	Of Special Notation	Nursing Assessments and Comments

Date and Time	Of Special Notation	Nursing Assessments and Comments

☐ *Practice Session*   At 9:00 P.M., you bring her fruit snack and a small glass of milk. She eats it all.

At 9:30 P.M., you spend a half-hour discussing how Mrs. Fox feels she is progressing with all the changes in her life. She is more optimistic and states, "You know, I'm beginning to feel as though I'll get through all this. I've almost got the injection bit down pat, and with a bit of help, maybe I'll get my diet straightened out too."

At 10:00 P.M., Mrs. Fox is quietly resting in bed.

Giving Verbal Nursing Reports

The verbal reports that you give concerning your patient can have a major influence on the overall health care that he receives. For example, look at the two verbal reports below. (Both examples are reports about the same patient.)

Verbal Nursing Report 1

"Mrs. J. has had her usual bad day. She is driving me crazy with her moaning and groaning about her back pain. I've given her everything I can, but she's still on the light all the time. . .and she even has her husband hopping around for every little request! The x-rays have been negative. This has been going on for 2 weeks! I wish they'd do something with her—I think she's just a crock, and this isn't a psychiatric unit. Her signs are stable, and intake and output okay. Good luck with her."

Verbal Nursing Report 2

"Mrs. J. seems to have had another bad day. She seems so uncomfortable. She states the pain medicine give very little relief, if any. Her husband has been very supportive and tries to help her, but nothing seems to work. The x-rays have been negative. It must be really hard to be here for 2 weeks without getting any better or finding out what's wrong. I wish we could do more for her. Her signs are stable and she's had 700 ml intake today. She should be encouraged to drink more during the evening."

If you compare the two examples above, you will probably notice the negativism and subjectivity of Report 1. The nurse has begun to pass on the word that "this patient is a crock." If continued, the attitude of the whole nursing staff can become negative. On the other hand, the nurse in Report 2 passes on the report of "I wish we could do more for her," which is a much more positive message.

The importance of verbal nursing reports cannot be underestimated. A good, clear verbal report can enhance the quality of nursing care and promote greater continuity. A poor, highly subjective report can create errors and confusion. For these reasons, you must be sure that you can give an organized, clear, objective nursing report.

Because the "end-of-the-shift" nursing report from a nurse who is going off duty to another nurse who is coming on duty is one of the most common forms of verbal nursing reports, let's take a look at some guidelines that you can follow when you give an end-of-the-shift report on your patients.

☐ *Guidelines*   *Giving an End-of-the-Shift Report*

☐ Begin by giving basic background information, including the following:

Name, room number, age, attending and consulting physicians

Date of admission, medical diagnoses, surgical procedures

Nursing diagnoses

EXAMPLE:

"Mrs. Ballard, in room 214 by the window, is a 35-year-old patient of Dr. Smith, with a consultation to Dr. Jones. She was admitted on 5/25 with pneumonia. She had a tracheostomy on 5/26. Her nursing diagnoses are Potential Ineffective Airway Clearance related to thick and copious secretions, Potential Impairment of Skin Integrity related to bed rest, and Anxiety related to new situation of hospitalization (has never been hospitalized before)."

☐ Give a general report on how the day went from the *patient's point of view*, rather than from your own point of view.

EXAMPLE:

Right: "Mr. Smith has not felt so well today."

Wrong: "I had a bad day with Mr. Smith."

☐ Don't be vague. Give specific observable data whenever possible.

EXAMPLES:

Right: "Mr. Smith has had an increase in his respiratory rate to 32/min. His heart rate is up to 122, and his temperature is 101."

Wrong: "Mr. Smith seems to be having respiratory difficulty."

Right: "I gave Mr. Smith 8 mg of morphine IM at 5:10 P.M. for incisional pain."

Wrong: "I gave Mr. Smith a pain med for his pain."

(continued)

☐ *Guidelines*

☐ When describing a problem, use the nursing process and describe assessment, diagnosis, planning, implementation, and evaluation in order to be sure that your report is organized.

EXAMPLE:

Right: "Mr. Smith complains of constipation. He hasn't had a bowel movement in 4 days. I gave him milk of magnesia and some prune juice this morning, but he still hasn't moved his bowels."

Wrong: "I gave Mr. Smith some milk of magnesia and some prune juice. He's constipated, and still has not moved his bowels. He hasn't gone in 4 days."

☐ If you make an inference, qualify your statement (*e.g.*, use a phrase such as "The patient seems to. . .").

EXAMPLE:

Right: "Mr. Smith seems withdrawn to me."

Wrong: "Mr. Smith has been withdrawn today."

☐ Describe the presence of all invasive medical treatments (*e.g.*, intravenous lines, Foley catheters, nasogastric tubes).

☐ Stress abnormal findings (*e.g.*, rales in the lungs, abnormal vital signs).

☐ Stress variations from routine (*e.g.*, "This patient will *not* have a preop medication").

☐ Describe the nursing care that has been done, including the following:

Assessment of vital signs

Focus assessment of current nursing diagnosis/collaborative problems

Patient activities (*e.g.*, "Ambulated well. . .")

Nursing interventions (*e.g.*, "Applied warm soaks. . .")

Measurement of intake and output (if applicable)

Medical interventions (*e.g.*, "Inserted central venous line. . .")

Diagnostic studies (*e.g.*, "Potassium was 3.8.")

☐ Describe the nursing care that has to be done, including the following:

Frequency of assessment of vital signs/specific assessment for potential complications (*e.g.*, "Observe for bleeding at catheter site.")

Diet

Patient activities

Nursing interventions

Medical treatments

Diagnostic studies

Ongoing Evaluation/Maintaining a Current Care Plan

Even before you get to a formal evaluation period, you should be performing ongoing evaluation of both patient care and your own nursing activities on a daily basis. You should be asking yourself two questions:

1. How is each of my patients responding to my nursing care?

2. How are my days going?

As you perform nursing interventions, you should be evaluating the daily progress of each of your patients. If a patient is not progressing, you should begin to examine factors that are impeding progress (this will be discussed in Chapter 6, Evaluation). If a patient is progressing well, you may want to consider if perhaps your patient could be doing more or moving at a quicker pace. You may even note that some of the problems that you originally identified have changed or disappeared. It is important to make changes that are obviously necessary before you get to a formal evaluation phase. All these changes should be documented on the nursing care plan so that all nurses who read the plan have a clear, up-to-date idea of the plan of care.

Revision of the care plan should include checking to be sure that the following information is up to date:

☐ Nursing diagnoses/collaborative problems

☐ Nursing orders (interventions)

☐ Goals/expected outcomes (with target dates for completion)

☐ Evaluation (reports on client progress)

(Modifying and revising the care plan will be further discussed in Chapter 6.)

In addition to evaluating patient progress, it is a good idea to take some time at the end of your day to determine if you, yourself, are having satisfactory days. Ask yourself the questions listed in Display 5-1.

Display 5-1. *Questions to Ask Yourself to Evaluate Your Work Day*

How has the day, in general, gone?

Have I completed everything I should have?

Have I been organized?

Have I been able to set priorities well?

What are some of the factors that have influenced how I have set priorities and organized my day?

(continued)

Display 5-1. *(Continued)*

Am I identifying both nursing diagnoses and collaborative problems for my patients?

How much time am I spending performing collaborative nursing interventions?

How much time am I spending implementing independent nursing interventions?

Could I be doing more?

Am I trying to do too much?

Are there changes I should make tomorrow?

☐ *Key Points*

Implementation

1. Implementation involves the following activities:

   Continuing assessment and data collection

   Performing nursing interventions (See Guidelines: Implementing [Performing] Nursing Interventions.)

   Documenting nursing care (See Guidelines: Charting Nurses' Notes.)

   Giving verbal nursing reports (See Guidelines: Giving an End-of-the-Shift Report.)

   Maintaining a current care plan

2. The nonsensical word "cwipat" can be used to remind you of the common tasks that should be accomplished before performing any nursing intervention. "Cwipat" stands for the following:

   C = *C*heck the orders and equipment.

   W = *W*ash your hands.

   I   = *I*dentify the patient.

   P = *P*rovide for safety and privacy.

   A = *A*ssess the problem.

   T = *T*ell the person or *T*each the person about what you're going to do.

3. You must continue to collect pertinent data and to assess the behaviors of your patient while you are performing nursing actions.

4. The verbal reports that you give concerning your patient can have a major influence on the overall health care that he receives.

5. Charting, or documentation of nursing care, is a legal requirement of all health-care systems.

6. Poor, illegible, or incomplete charting may impede nursing care because

□ *Key Points*

it will be more difficult to recognize significant changes in health status without clear documentation of client activities and behaviors.

7. Good, factually descriptive nursing notes will enhance patient care because they will communicate the pertinent aspects of the client's health care and help others to assess patterns of client responses.

8. Nursing care plans are useless unless they are kept up to date.

9. Part of the implementation phase involves ongoing evaluation of both your patient and yourself. (See Display 5-1.)

□ *Bibliography*

American Nurses' Association: Standards of Nursing Practice. Kansas City, MO, American Nurses' Association, 1973

Carpenito L: Nursing Diagnosis: Application to Clinical Practice. Philadelphia, JB Lippincott, 1983

Eggland E: Charting: How and when to document your daily care. Nursing '80 10:38–43, 1980

Gordon M: Nursing Diagnosis: Process and Application. New York, McGraw-Hill, 1982

Griffith J, Christensen P: Nursing Process: Application of Theories, Frameworks and Models. St Louis, CV Mosby, 1982

Kerr A: Nurses' notes: That's where the goodies are. Nursing '75 5:34–41, 1975

Kozier B, Erb G: Fundamentals of Nursing: Concepts and Process. Menlo Park, CA, Addison-Wesley, 1979

Potter P, Perry A: Fundamentals of Nursing Concepts: Concepts, Process, and Practice. St Louis, CV Mosby, 1985

Van Hoozer H, Ruther L, Craft M: Introduction to Charting. Philadelphia, JB Lippincott, 1982

- ☑ Establishing outcome criteria
- ☑ Evaluating goal achievement
- ☑ Identifying variables affecting goal achievement
- ☑ Modifying the plan of care/ terminating care

6

Evaluation

Standard VII: *The client's/patient's progress or lack of progress toward goal achievement is determined by the client/patient and the nurse.*

Standard VIII: *The client's/patient's progress or lack of progress toward goal achievement directs reassessment, reordering of priorities, new goal setting, and revision of the plan of nursing care.**

**Abstracted from Standards—Nursing Practice. Copyright American Nurses' Association, 1973

☐ *Glossary*   ***Nursing audit***   The thorough investigation designed to identify, examine, or verify the performance of certain specified aspects of nursing care through the use of established professional standards (Potter and Perry, 1985)

Quality assurance program   A program designed to perform audits and to establish standards of client care that will demonstrate high-quality health care

Evaluation is the fifth step of the nursing process. It is during this phase that you will be determining how well your plan of nursing care has worked. That is, you will have to determine if the client has achieved the goals of the plan of care. Although evaluation is often called the "final step" of the nursing process, you may have noticed that, to a certain degree, you actually have been evaluating your plan of care all along. During each of the preceding steps of the nursing process, you began early evaluation when you continued to reassess your client, to rearrange priorities, and to observe client behaviors and responses. However, it is during this fifth step that you should complete a thorough reassessment of the entire plan of care. This thorough evaluation is necessary to help you to determine if you have indeed designed the best plan of care possible for this specific individual. It will also help you to identify the necessary changes that will further improve the plan of care.

Evaluation involves the following activities:

☐ Establishing the criteria for evaluation
☐ Evaluating goal achievement
☐ Assessing variables affecting goal achievement
☐ Modifying the plan of care / terminating nursing care

Establishing the Criteria for Evaluation/Evaluating Goal Achievement

Ideally the criteria that you establish for evaluation will be the same as the goals or outcomes that you have identified during the planning phase. That is, you established goals for your client during the planning phase, and now you must decide how well he has achieved the goals. As discussed in Chapter 4, some institutions will have already established certain outcome criteria for given problems. Given that you established goals that were congruent with the standard outcome criteria of the facility where you are working, the criteria for evaluation will be the goals that you established.

In order to evaluate goal achievement, you will have to compare your client's actions or behaviors with the goals that you set forth in the planning phase. For example, you may have established the goal of "will walk a half mile in 10 minutes by July 28th." On July 28th you should evaluate whether the client can walk a half mile in 10 minutes. If he cannot, how far can he walk in 10 minutes? Is he close to his goal? How well does he walk the half mile? Is he very tired when he does it, or does he do it with relative ease? Because the goal is the ultimate aim of the plan of care, evaluating goal achievement is a major part of the evaluation process. Display 6-1 lists suggested steps to help you to evaluate goal achievement.

Display 6-1.   *Steps for Evaluating Goal Achievement*

1. List the goals (outcome criteria) that you have set forth in the planning phase.

   EXAMPLE:

   "Will walk unassisted the length of the hall by 7/3."

2. Assess what the client is able to do in relation to the goals.

   EXAMPLE:

   "Can walk unassisted the length of the hall, but he becomes a little unsteady toward the end of the walk."

3. Compare what the client is able to do with what you have set as his goal and ask the following questions:

   Has the goal been *completely* met? Can the client do *everything* set forth by the goal with the conditions set forth by the goal? How *well* does he perform the activities set forth by the goal?

   Has the goal been *partially* met? Is the client able to do only some of the activities set forth by the goals? Is he able to do the activities, but not with good proficiency? Does the client seem to be struggling to achieve the goal?

   Has the goal *not been met* at all?

4. Discuss the goals with the client. Encourage him to verbalize his feelings about whether or not he has achieved the goals.

5. If all the goals have been easily achieved, are you moving too slowly, or are you going at just the right pace? Could you be doing more? Discuss this with the client, his family, and health-care team.

6. If the goals have only been partially met, or not met at all, gather data to determine what has gone wrong.

   Have short-term goals been met?

   Are the goals realistic for this individual?

   Does the client feel these goals are important?

(continued)

Display 6-1. *(Continued)*

> What does the client feel is important?
>
> Can the client identify anything that he feels may be slowing him down?
>
> Can you identify anything that may be slowing him down?
>
> Has the plan of care indeed been implemented, or have some actions been omitted?

7. Record your findings. Write an evaluation statement that includes how well goals have been achieved. (This is usually written in the column marked "evaluation" or "progress report" on the nursing care plan.)

Assessing the Variables Affecting Goal Achievement

Once you have determined how well you and the client are achieving your goals, it is important to gather information to help you to determine what are the variables that are affecting your success or failure. What are the factors that are helping you to achieve goals, and what are the factors that may be impeding your progress? Determining these "strengths and weaknesses" requires a full reassessment of the client's health state. This includes gathering data concerning his physical and psychological well-being, as well as his physical and social environment. You need to reassess your client to determine the following:

☐ Are the problems the same as originally defined?

☐ Are they more complicated than originally described?

☐ Have new problems arisen?

☐ Are the interventions you have chosen appropriate?

☐ What motivates or discourages this individual?

The client himself is often the key person who can identify factors that are either helping or hindering him in goal achievement, and you should ask him whether he felt the plan was a good plan for him. Let him know that this information could help other people in similar situations.

You, too, will have to apply your nursing knowledge to identify some of these factors. For example, you may find that a client who has just been diagnosed as having diabetes is not achieving a goal of "will verbalize how insulin affects the blood sugar level." Instead, the client seems quiet and disinterested. You will need to gather data to learn why the client is withdrawn and disinterested. Perhaps he has not yet accepted that he has diabetes and needs some time and interventions to help him accept his disease before he can motivate himself to learn about diabetes.

Modifying the Plan of Care

Once you have determined whether you have set realistic goals and identified some variables that may be affecting goal achievement, you are now ready to modify the plan of care. You may need to establish new goals, identify new interventions, or change the environment or timing of interventions. Modifying a plan of care requires an open, inquisitive mind. It is a good idea to plan a conference with both the client and other health-care professionals who are involved in the plan of care so that you get input concerning necessary changes from as many qualified people as possible.

Display 6-2 lists suggested steps to help you to modify your plan of care.

Display 6-2.   *Steps for Modifying the Plan of Care*

1. Gather data to determine if any new problems have arisen and if your original nursing diagnoses and collaborative problems are still appropriate. Look for gaps or incongruities in the original assessment data that were documented. Seek to fill in the gaps and clarify incongruous facts by performing a full reassessment of the client.

2. Delete nursing diagnoses and collaborative problems that are not appropriate. Add any that are new.

3. Examine your list of nursing diagnoses and collaborative problems and set new priorities if necessary.

4. If you decide that the diagnoses and problems that you have identified are accurate and current, examine each established goal and ask the following questions:

   Is each goal derived specifically for a separate nursing diagnosis or collaborative problem?

   Are the goals realistic for this individual?

   Is the time frame for goal achievement realistic?

   Do the goals reflect individual capabilities and preferences of the client?

6. Change those goals that are unrealistic. (Either determine a more realistic goal, or set a new time frame for goal achievement.) Change those goals that do not reflect the individual preferences of your client. (Rewrite the goals to reflect his individual capabilities and preferences.)

7. Delete goals that are inappropriate, and add new goals if new problems or diagnoses have been identified.

(continued)

Display 6-2. *(Continued)*

8. Examine the interventions that have been identified for each of the appropriate goals, and ask the following:

Is the written plan of nursing interventions being put into action consistently?

Do the interventions promote individual client strengths?

Is the timing of interventions appropriate, or should they be rearranged?

Is the environment conducive to performing the activities necessary for the interventions?

Are the interventions producing the desired responses?

What are some additional factors or interventions that might help to produce the desired response?

9. Change or delete interventions that are inappropriate, and add any new interventions that have been identified.

10. Incorporate factors that contribute to your client's successful goal achievement, and delete or minimize factors that may be impeding progress.

11. Set new target dates for reevaluation.

Terminating Nursing Care

If you have achieved all your goals and have not identified new problems, you have achieved the ultimate aim of nursing care: terminating the plan of care and allowing the person full control over his own health. When you know you are ready to terminate nursing care, you can really feel as though you and the patient have met with success. Even though the actual act of terminating happens during the evaluation phase of the nursing process, terminating (or discharging) is something that you should be talking about from the time of your first encounter with the patient. Some nurses view discharge as a sort of "present" the patient gets on the day he goes home (*e.g.*, "Guess what, *today* is the day you get to go home!"). It would be better if we discussed discharge as a *right* that will soon belong to the patient. During the entire time that you are delivering nursing care, you should be discussing "when you are discharged" whenever appropriate. This helps to prepare the patient from the beginning that the whole goal of nursing care should be that of making him as independent as possible.

Terminating nursing care involves a full assessment of how the patient plans to manage his health on his own.

Written and verbal instructions for treatments, medications, and activities should be given to the patient to take home. Signs and symptoms of any possible future problems should be discussed, written down on paper, and given to the patient to take home. Important telephone numbers and services that are available to the patient should also be discussed and written down. The patient and his family should be able to verbalize the types of problems they should be avoiding and preventing, the correct management of their specific problems, and the resources that they may be planning to use to improve their health. Most health-care facilities have their own discharge planning and discharge instruction forms that must be completed before discharge, and you should become familiar with each of these.

Nursing Audits and Quality Assurance

It would be inappropriate to conclude a chapter on evaluation of nursing care without a brief discussion of nursing audits and quality assurance. Many health-care facilities have established programs for quality assurance that are designed to evaluate nursing care and to identify factors that either promote or impede good health care. Factors that are identified as being essential for good health care become the accepted standards of care for the facility. Once the standards are identified, a nursing audit can be employed to evaluate patient care. In order to perform an audit, a thorough investigation of patient records must be accomplished to determine the quality of care in relation to the accepted standards. For example, the quality assurance program of a given hospital may have determined a standard that all patients admitted to any patient care area must have a useful, documented nursing care plan within the first 24 hours after admission. In order to see if these standards are being met, an audit would be performed, and patient charts would be reviewed to determine if useful care plans were documented within 24 hours of admission. Obviously, the key to a successful audit and quality assurance program is that of having an accurate, complete system of documentation of patient care.

Quality assurance programs and nursing audits provide a vehicle for documentation of high standards of nursing care to be used by all nurses as a basis for implementing high-quality nursing care.

☐ *Key Points*   *Evaluation*

1. The fifth step of the nursing process, evaluation, involves a complete reassessment of the entire plan of nursing care.

2. Evaluation involves the following activities:

    Establishing outcome criteria

    Evaluating goal achievement

    Assessing variables affecting goal achievement

    Modifying plan of care / terminating nursing care

3. Whether a goal has been achieved should be determined by both the client and the nurse.

(*continued*)

☐ *Key Points*

4. To determine goal achievement, you must ascertain what the client can do in relation to the goals set forth during the planning phase of the nursing process (see Display 6-1).

5. Evaluation involves assessing what factors may be contributing to the success of the plan, and what factors may be impeding your progress.

6. Modifying the plan of care involves revising the plan of care to begin a new plan of care that reflects the necessary changes that were noted by full reassessment of the nursing care plan (see Display 6-2).

7. Terminating nursing care, or discharge planning, should begin as early in the plan of care as possible. For example, when appropriate, include discussions of "when you are discharged" even if the discharge date is a long way off.

☐ *Bibliography*

American Nurses' Association: Standards of Nursing Practice. Kansas City, MO, American Nurses' Association, 1973

Carpenito L: Nursing Diagnosis: Application to Clinical Practice. Philadelphia, JB Lippincott, 1983

Duke University Hospital Nursing Services: Duke Guidelines for Nursing Care: Process and Outcome, 2nd ed. Philadelphia, JB Lippincott, 1983

Gordon M: Nursing Diagnosis: Process and Application. New York, McGraw-Hill, 1982

Griffith J, Christensen P: Nursing Process: Application of Theories, Frameworks and Models. St Louis, CV Mosby, 1982

Kozier B, Erb G: Fundamentals of Nursing: Concepts and Process. Menlo Park, CA, Addison-Wesley, 1979

Potter P, Perry A: Fundamentals of Nursing Concepts: Concepts, Process, and Practice. St Louis, CV Mosby, 1985

Spotts S: A nursing diagnosis taxonomy for quality assurance and reimbursement. Pennsylvania Nurse 36:5, 1981

Van Hoozer H, Ruther L, Craft M: Introduction to Charting. Philadelphia, JB Lippincott, 1982

Warren J: Accountability and nursing diagnosis. J Nurs Adm 13:34–37, 1981

Suggested Answers to Practice Sessions

Note

When you check your answers with the suggested answers on the following pages, please remember that these are *suggested* answers. In some cases, you may find that you have somewhat different answers than those that are given by the suggested answers. This does not necessarily mean that your answer is wrong. It is difficult to present a clear, concise case history on paper—too often there is room for varied interpretation by the reader. These sessions are meant to *provide practice* in the thinking process necessary to complete the steps of the nursing process, and these are the *suggested* answers, not the *only* answers. Check with your instructor if you have a question.

Chapter 1: Nursing Process Overview (page 15)

1. The nursing process plan focuses on human responses, while the medical treatment plan focuses on disease. The nursing process plan is more likely to change on a day-to-day basis as human responses change. The medical treatment plan is more likely to stay the same for longer periods of time. The nursing process also deals more with families and groups than does the average medical treatment plan.

2. *Assessment:* Gathering data for the purpose of identifying actual and potential health problems

    Diagnosis: Analyzing data and identifying the exact nature of a health problem

    Planning: Establishing goals and determining nursing interventions

    Implementation: Putting the plan into action

    Evaluation: Measuring goal achievement, determining factors that influenced patient care, and terminating or modifying the plan of care as indicated

3. Provides for organized nursing care

    Prevents omissions and unnecessary repetitions

    Provides for better communication

    Focuses on the individual's unique human response

    Promotes flexibility in giving individualized nursing care

    Encourages participation on the part of the patient

    Helps nurses to gain satisfaction by getting results

Chapter 2: Assessment (page 34)

The Nursing Interview

1. Making open-ended questions
    a. "Describe how you feel."

   b. "How was your dinner?"

   c. "How does being here make you feel?"

   d. "Describe what it feels like."

   e. "Tell me about your relationship with your wife."

2. Clarifying ideas by using reflection and making open-ended questions

   a. "You've been sick off and on for a month? Describe what the sickness is like."

   b. "Nothing ever goes right for you? Give some examples of what you mean."

   c. "So, you have a pain in your side that is intermittent. Explain how it feels and what you mean by 'comes and goes'."

   d. "...A funny feeling? Describe the feeling."

   e. "You feel weak all over? Give me some examples of things that make you feel weak."

Organizing the Nursing Physical Assessment   (page 38)

Case History I

1. Mental status

   Vital signs

   Pain

   Fluid and electrolyte balance

2. Interview Mrs. Laird about symptoms/concerns.

   Ask about abdominal symptoms (pain, nausea, vomiting, bowel movements).

   Perform abdominal assessment. (Assess for presence of bowel sounds, distention, tenderness.)

   Assess fluid intake and output. (Assess for dehydration.)

   Read medical and nursing records (care plan, nurses' notes, progress notes, lab studies, x-ray reports).

Case History II

1. Vital signs

   Respiratory status (lung sounds, cough, mucus production, whether he has been smoking since surgery, method for coughing)

   Surgical incision/heparin lock

   When last analgesic was administered

   Intake and output (Assess for adquate hydration.)

2. Interview Mr. Daniels about symptoms/concerns.

Perform an abdominal assessment. Examine incision.

Auscultate lungs.

Have the patient demonstrate coughing and deep breathing (examine sputum).

Read medical and nursing records (care plan, nurses' notes, progress reports, lab studies, x-ray reports).

Subjective and Objective Data   (page 40)

Case History I

1. 51 years old

No pain

Feels better

Feels relieved

2. Lab study results

Talking slowly

Frequent sighing

Vital signs

Case History II

1. 33 years old

Mother of two

"I can't believe I have diabetes."

"I don't think I can change my eating habits."

Feels fine, but tired lately

Increased urination

2. Weight: 190 lb

Blood sugar: 144

Vital signs

Identifying Cues and Inferences   (page 43)

1. All the subjective and objective data listed under Mr. Michaels in the previous practice session.

2. Physical condition improving

Seems depressed

3. All the subjective and objective data listed under Mrs. Rochester in the previous practice session

4. Seems reluctant to admit she has diabetes

   Seems anxious concerning effects of diabetes and changes in life-style (*e.g.*, eating habits)

   May be angry about diagnosis

Validating Assessment Data   *(page 45)*

1.

Certainly Valid	*Probably Valid*	*Possibly Valid*
Lab studies	51 years old	Feels relieved
Talking slowly	No pain	
Frequent sighing	Feels better	
	Vital signs	

2. Compare stated age with birthdate.

   Ask probing questions to describe comfort state (*e.g.*, "Are you *sure* you don't have any discomfort at all?").

   Observe for nonverbal signs of discomfort (*e.g.*, rubbing hand on chest).

   Spend quality time with Mr. Michaels discussing how he feels physically and psychologically.

   Recheck vital signs if you are concerned that they are inaccurate.

3.

Certainly Valid	*Probably Valid*	*Possibly Valid*
Weight: 190 lb	33 years old	Angry about having diabetes
Blood sugar: 144	Mother of two	May be denying that she has diabetes
	Anxious	
	Feels tired	
	Increased urination	

4. Compare stated age with birthdate.

   Measure time and amount of urine output.

   Spend quality time discussing feelings and concerns about changes in life-style.

Organizing Assessment Data   *(page 50)*

Case History I

If you used Maslow's hierarchy of needs:

Physiological needs: 5,6,7,9,11,12,13,14

Safety/security needs: 10

Love and belonging needs: 2,4,8

Self-esteem needs: 3,8,11,13

Self-actualization needs: 3

Case History II *(page 51)*

If you used Gordon's functional health patterns:

Health-perception–health-management pattern: 10,11

Nutritional-metabolic pattern: 1,5,6,9,13,14,16

Elimination pattern: 9

Activity/exercise pattern: 2

Cognitive-perceptual pattern: 12

Sleep-rest pattern: 8

Self-perception–self-concept pattern: 1,2,3

Role-relationship pattern: 2,3,7

Sexuality-reproductive pattern: 1,2

Coping-stress-tolerance pattern: 7,12

Value-belief pattern: 4

Chapter 3: Diagnosis *(page 65)*

Nursing Diagnoses/Collaborative Problems

1. CP		9. ND	
2. ND		10. CP	
3. ND		11. CP	
4. CP		12. ND	
5. ND		13. ND	
6. ND		14. CP	
7. CP		15. CP	
8. CP			

Using the PES Format *(page 71)*

1. Impaired Gas Exchange related to smoking as manifested by chronic cough productive of mucus, constant smoking, elevated CO_2.

2. Alteration in Nutrition: Less Than Body Requirements related to loss of appetite as manifested by 10-lb weight loss and weight that is 15 lb less than the recommended weight

3. Impaired Physical Mobility related to inability to move lower limbs as manifested by inability to move both lower legs and limited passive range of motion in lower joints

4. Potential for Injury related to blindness and environmental hazards as manifested by statements that he falls and bumps himself all the time and large bruise on forehead

Writing Diagnostic Statements for Potential and Possible Nursing Diagnoses *(page 75)*

1. Possible Ineffective Individual Coping related to problems with his girlfriend and possibly related to confinement to bed

2. Potential Fluid Volume Deficit related to insufficient fluid intake

3. Potential Ineffective Airway Clearance related to history of smoking and recent general anesthesia

4. Possible Sexual Dysfunction possibly related to recent hysterectomy, or possibly related to poor relationship with her husband

Identifying Correctly Stated Nursing Diagnoses *(page 78)*

The following are correct: 5, 6, 8, 9, 13, 15

Identifying Nursing Diagnoses and Collaborative Problems *(page 85)*

Case History I (Mrs. Goode)

Nursing Diagnoses:

Potential for Injury related to dizziness

Potential Alteration in Patterns of Urinary Elimination related to inability to use bed pan

Fear related to hospitalization as manifested by statements of fear of hospitals and needles

Possible Alteration in Family Processes related to Mrs. Goode's illness

Collaborative Problems:

Potential Complication: increased intracranial pressure

Potential Complication: phlebitis or tissue injury at intravenous site

Case History II (Mr. Northe)

Nursing Diagnoses:

Alteration in Bowel Elimination: Constipation related to inactivity as manifested by no bowel movement in 5 days

Impaired Physical Mobility related to prescribed bed rest as manifested by prescribed bed rest

Potential Ineffective Individual Coping related to prescribed bed rest

Possible Fear of Death related to brother's death under the same circumstances

Possible Spiritual Distress related to uncertainty of cardiac condition and threat to life

Impairment of Skin Integrity as manifested by red pressure areas on both heels

Collaborative Problems:

Potential complication:

Cardiac arrhythmias

Congestive heart failure

Pulmonary edema

Atelectasis

Oliguria

Fluid overload per IV

Phlebitis, tissue injury at IV site

Chapter 4: Planning

Writing Expected Goals/Outcomes   (page 102)

1. List, identify, describe, verbalize, demonstrate, report

2. The following are *incorrect:*

   a. The verb is not measurable.

   c. Nonspecific. How will we measure what is meant by "will improve"?

   f. No time criterion. Verb is not measurable and observable.

   h. No time criterion. Verb is not measurable and observable.

   j. Verb is not measurable.

Establishing Client Goals/Expected Outcomes   (page 104)

1. After increasing roughage intake, Mrs. Pierce will report having one soft, formed bowel movement every 1 to 2 days, beginning Thursday.

2. After Diane begins performing daily tooth brushing, flossing,

and gum care, her gums will be pink and healthy looking (by 10/28).

3. When observed, the skin around Mr. Culp's incision will be clean, with no signs of redness or irritation.

4. After instruction, Mrs. Sovosky will correctly express needs by using flash cards (by 4/26).

5. After a visit by the chaplain, Heidi will verbalize that it is "OK with God" if she is unable to go to daily Mass and that knowing this makes her feel more peaceful.

6. Mrs. O'Dell will demonstrate how to feed herself with the use of padded spoons by 5/9.

7. Mr. Noll will stop smoking or reduce smoking and/or report to the nurse if he develops respiratory symptoms.

8. Mrs. Bell will eat three balanced meals every day with a caloric intake of 2000.

9. Mr. Roberts will not be disturbed, but will be observed sleeping soundly for periods of 4 hours at night beginning tonight.

10. Jane will report ability to void at least 200 ml without pain or urgency.

Domains of Expected Outcomes   *(page 106)*

1. a. Cognitive and psychomotor
   b. Cognitive
   c. Affective
   d. Cognitive
   e. Cognitive and psychomotor
   f. Psychomotor
   g. Affective
   h. Psychomotor and cognitive
   i. Cognitive
   j. Cognitive, psychomotor, and affective

2. a. View film on infant nutrition and formula feedings on 4/5.

   Describe the steps involved in preparing and sterilizing formula on 4/5.

   Demonstrate preparing and sterilizing baby formula on 4/6.

   b. Read the procedure for sterilization, and clarify any questions with primary nurse on 5/1.

   Verbalize the reasons for sterilization on 5/10.

c. Discuss with primary nurse on 2/2 how patient feels about going home.

d. Attend the diabetic class on nutrition on 10/11.

Discuss with primary nurse the relationship between blood sugar levels and eating certain foods on 10/11.

Review printed diet restrictions on 10/12.

e. Attend the group diabetic class on insulin administration and monitoring of blood sugar levels on 7/28.

View teaching filmstrips on insulin administration and the monitoring of blood sugar on 7/29.

Observe the nurse demonstrating the correct procedures for insulin administration and for testing blood sugar level on 7/30.

Practice insulin self-administration based on morning blood sugar readings beginning 7/31.

f. After instruction by physical therapy on 12/2, Mr. Roberts will begin practicing walking with a cane, gradually increasing how far he walks until he can walk the length of the hall (by 12/7).

g. On 1/14 discuss with Mrs. Bell the importance of verbalizing when she is worried or concerned.

h. On 3/2, have Debbie observe the correct technique for postural drainage, then encourage her to ask questions for clarification.

On 3/3 and 3/4 have Debbie practice performing postural drainage under close supervision.

i. Teach Matt the signs and symptoms of hypoglycemia using the "diabetic game" on 2/5.

Informally quiz Matt on the signs and symptoms on 2/6, and reinforce information that he does not seem to know.

j. Watch film on balanced nutrition on 11/11.

Discuss how Jimmy can make time to cook and eat breakfast.

Assist Jimmy to incorporate favorite foods into a balanced diet.

Determining Nursing Interventions for Nursing Diagnoses *(page 112)*

1. Assess skin integrity, especially over bony prominences, with each position change.

Assess protein and vitamin C intake.

Develop (and post at bedside) a q 2 hour turning schedule that enlists the client's maximal participation.

Massage bony prominences with Alpha Keri lotion with position changes.

Keep an air mattress on the bed. Keep sheets clean, dry, and unwrinkled.

2. *Preoperatively:*

After demonstrating the correct procedure for coughing and deep breathing with incisional splinting, assess the patient's and family's knowledge of these procedures via return demonstration.

Postoperatively:

Assess for incisional pain. Medicate p.r.n. as indicated.

Auscultate lungs bilaterally, and record findings.

Assist client with coughing and deep breathing q 2 hours the day of surgery and first postoperative day.

Teach the client the importance of position changes, early ambulation, and coughing and deep breathing.

3. Continue to assess daily bowel habits.

Teach the client the relationship between exercise, diet, fluid intake, and normal bowel elimination.

Develop with the client a specific plan for gradually increasing daily activity (*e.g.,* using stairs instead of elevator, or walking briskly) and for increasing dietary intake of roughage and fluids (especially water).

4. Assess incisional dressing with each post-operative change.

When changing the dressing, assess the incision for signs of healing. Report any signs of infection: redness, swelling, drainage with foul odor.

Utilize sterile technique when changing the dressing: cleanse the incision with betadine and cover with a sterile dressing.

Teach the client how to care for the healing incision at home, including how to detect and manage complications.

5. Primary nurse should discuss with client key factors of his hospitalization that are making the client feel powerless.

Determine with client what aspects of his hospitalization he feels that he is able to control.

Alert the nursing staff to give client control in as many of these areas as possible.

Teach the client that his body and his health are his own and that he has the right to make autonomous decisions about his health care. Provide the knowledge base that makes this possible. Support him in physician–client interactions.

Writing Nursing Orders   *(page 122)*

1. Develop a turning schedule for q 2 hour position changes and post the schedule at bedside.

   Assess the client's understanding of the need for position changes and ability/willingness to help. Assess the family's ability/desire to assist with position changes.

   Turn the client q 2 hours, noting any changes in skin integrity, massaging bony prominences, and providing for good body alignment.

2. Assess what fluid preferences the client has and order these fluids for the unit. Keep preferred fluids at the bedside at all times.

   Utilize all client interactions to encourage fluid intake. Each shift should be responsible for:

7–3 = 1800 ml	3–11 = 1000 ml	11–7 = 200 ml

   Teach the client the importance of increasing his fluid intake. Assess his understanding of the need to force fluids and his willingness to do so.

   Tell the person the goal for fluid intake, and have him record what he drinks.

3. Utilize all patient interactions (nursing rounds, bath time, treatments, etc.) to develop a trusting nurse–patient relationship. Utilize empathic behaviors that express genuine caring.

   Encourage the person to express her feelings by using open-ended questions (*e.g.*, "It must be hard to lie there all afternoon with nothing to do but think. What are you thinking about?").

   If one or more nurses establish a good rapport with this patient, assign them frequently to her care.

   Attempt to determine why it is difficult for this individual to express her feelings. Share with her the positive benefits of expression, as well as the potential negative consequences of holding things in.

4. Assess the client's normal pattern of bowel elimination. Note any stimuli to bowel elimination (*e.g.*, jogging, morning coffee, etc.).

   Teach the client the relationship between adequate fluid/roughage intake and exercise and reguar bowel elimination.

   Teach the client the negative consequences of repeatedly ignoring the urge to defecate.

   Teach the client the harmful effects of prolonged use of laxatives and enemas.

   Instruct the client to record his daily bowel elimination, noting diet, exercise, and use of laxatives.

5. Assist patient out of bed to chair for a half hour, at 10 A.M. and 8 P.M. Provide two pillows for his back, and stool for feet. Leave call bell attached to R arm of chair.

Chapter 5: Implementation

Charting Nurses' Notes   (page 140)

Date and Time	Of Special Notation	Nursing Comments
11/22/85 8:30 AM		Sitting OOB in chair. Seems to be wheezing more than usual—using accessory muscles of the chest. Denies increased difficulty breathing.
8:40 AM	Reg 97–130–30 $\frac{170}{94}$	Respiratory rate unchanged, but he is more restless & confused (doesn't know he's in the hospital). _____ J. LeFevre, RN
8:45 AM	O₂ started @ 2liters/min per cannula	Assisted back to bed. Siderails ↑._____ Still wheezing and appears in distress. Dr. Payne notified. _____ J. LeFevre, RN
9 AM	Exam by Dr. Payne	Condition unchanged._____ J. LeFevre, RN
9:10 AM	ABGs drawn by Lab	Pressure to puncture site applied for 5 minutes—no bleeding. _____ J. LeFevre, RN
9:15 AM	Resp Therapist here for IPPB Rx._____	Coughed up large amount of thick white mucus. _____ J. LeFevre, RN
9:35 AM		Lungs more clear. He is no longer confused. Able to take a few sips of water. J. LeFevre, RN Much improved. Assisted OOB to chair.
10 AM	P-110 R-28	_____ J. LeFevre, RN

Case II (Mrs. Fox)

Date and Time	Of Special Notation	Nursing Assessments and Comments
6/14/86 5 PM		Assisted to give her own insulin._____ She contaminated needle and did not notice it. Reinforced the importance of maintaining sterile technique. _____ J. Koonce, RN
8 PM		Ate all of her dinner tonight, but she states that she is "dying for a chocolate bar"—she states that following a diabetic diet will be impossible. Discussed possibility of talking c̄ dietitian re: changes in diet. _____ J. Koonce, RN
8:30 PM		Encouraged to do things to get her mind off of food. Called a friend to chat. ___ J. Koonce, RN
9 PM		Offered her fruit & milk snack—ate it all & drank milk. _____ J. Koonce, RN
9:30–9:55		Spent time discussing her feelings about all the changes that she has to make because of diabetes. Is more optimistic now. _ J. Koonce, RN
10 PM		Resting quietly in bed. _____ J. Koonce, RN

Appendix

North American Nursing Diagnosis Association
Diagnosis Review Cycle*

The North American Nursing Diagnosis Association (NANDA), in an effort to meet its purpose "to develop, refine, and promote a taxonomy of nursing diagnostic terminology of general use to professional nurses" has developed a formal cycle of diagnosis review to enable the process of incorporation of new diagnoses submitted by interested parties. This process is cyclic in character, assuring continuous development and refinement of the taxonomy.

Step 1. Receipt of diagnoses: Diagnoses may be entered into the review cycle either on the initiative of NANDA or others.

A. NANDA initiates this process by soliciting diagnoses, advertising of their interest in diagnoses, publishing their guidelines for submission, and responding to inquiries concerning such guidelines.

B. Individual nurses or nurse groups initiate this process by submitting a diagnosis for review. When a submission is received by NANDA, it is initially reviewed for compliance with submission guidelines. Those submissions which involve only a suggested name or are only partially developed are returned to the person submitting the recommendation with a request for completion as described in the guidelines. Those submissions which meet criteria of the guidelines then enter the review process. The person submitting the suggested diagnosis receives a copy of the description of the Diagnosis Review Cycle at this time, to facilitate an understanding of NANDA's policies and procedures.

Step 2. Diagnoses enter the public domain: NANDA formally recognizes all diagnoses under review as part of the public domain. As such, any diagnosis submitted for review is briefly reported in the *NANDA Newsletter* when it enters the review cycle. Persons submitting diagnoses are advised of this fact and are asked to indicate in writing their acceptance of this policy on a form provided by NANDA.

It is recognized, however, that individuals have often invested considerable time and energy in an effort to delineate one or more diagnoses. Therefore, the publication of a diagnoses entering the review cycle will include the name of the person(s) submitting this diagnosis, assuring them of recognition of their efforts. This will also improve networking and communication among members actively engaged in exploring common or comparable diagnoses.

* Reprinted with permission of the North American Nursing Diagnosis Association. New diagnoses should be mailed to NANDA, St. Louis University Department of Nursing, 3525 Caroline Street, St. Louis, MO 63104.

Step 3. Diagnoses are reviewed by clinical technical task forces: The NANDA Diagnosis Review Committee (DRC) is charged with the task of reviewing proposed diagnoses and recommending their acceptance, modification, or rejection to the NANDA Board. This committee's work is guided by the advice and critique of clinical/technical task forces who review diagnoses.

A.   Each diagnosis accepted for review is assigned by the Chairperson of the Diagnosis Review Committee (DRC) to a member of that committee. This person serves as a primary or lead reviewer of the diagnosis and the Chairperson of the Clinical/Technical Review Task Force which will review the diagnosis.

B.   The Clinical/Technical Review Task Force is a panel created to review a specific diagnosis based on individual clinical and technical expertise. Task force members are drawn not only from NANDA membership, but also from expert groups in organizations such as the Canadian Nurses' Association and the American Nurses' Association. NANDA board members who do not serve on the Diagnosis Review Committee (DRC) are ineligible to serve on these task forces. Task forces are created as needed and appropriate by the Diagnosis Review Committee (DRC).

C.   Members of the various task forces receive diagnoses for critique and review with an evaluation form provided. This evaluation form enables reviewers to assess the degree to which the diagnosis submitted meets the criteria of the submission guidelines. Task force members are given two to four weeks to respond to a request for a review. These reviews are forwarded to the primary reviewer.

D.   Based on task force members' advice and comments, the primary reviewer prepares a diagnosis proposal for each diagnosis. These are presented at a meeting of the Diagnosis Review Committee.

Step 4. Diagnoses are reviewed by the NANDA Diagnosis Review Committee: The Diagnosis Review Committee convenes to review, discuss, and take action on the proposals for new diagnoses prepared by the primary reviewers of the Clinical/Technical Task Forces. Three possible outcomes emerge from this process.

A.   The DRC accepts the proposed diagnosis or makes minor changes, or

B.   The DRC substantively alters the diagnosis as submitted by the original proposer, based on reviewer advice. The DRC then accepts the proposed diagnosis, or

C.   The DRC rejects the diagnosis and identifies specific reasons for the rejection. In this case, the original proposer of the diagnosis is provided with specific recommendations for improvement.

The DRC notifies the original proposer of the diagnosis of their action at this time. They concurrently forward their recommendations to the NANDA Board.

Step 5. Diagnoses are reviewed by the NANDA Board: The NANDA Board receives the recommendations of the DRC and convenes to review, discuss, and take action on the DRC recommendations. Once more, three possible outcomes emerge from this process.

A. The Board accepts the DRC recommendation, or

B. The Board returns the diagnosis to the DRC with comments for revision and recommendations for change, or

C. The Board rejects the DRC recommendation and identifies specific reasons for the rejection.

The DRC then notifies the original proposer of the Board's action and prepares accepted diagnoses for General Assembly review and comment.

Step 6. Diagnoses are reviewed by the General Assembly: The General Assembly has the authority to review and comment on proposed diagnoses for the DRC's actions prior to the submission to the membership for acceptance. The DRC prepares proposed diagnoses for this review and comment. The DRC therefore engages in the following activities:

A. The DRC groups the diagnoses as possible or appropriate for General Assembly review.

B. The DRC structures time for review and comment by the General Assembly during the National Conference, advising the original proposer of the diagnosis of this action.

C. The DRC develops policies, procedures, and protocols for General Assembly review and comment and conducts these sessions accordingly.

D. The DRC collects General Assembly comments and incorporates these into proposed diagnoses as appropriate and feasible.

E. The DRC reports these changes to the Board.

Step 7. Diagnoses are voted upon by the NANDA membership: The DRC prepares diagnoses for a NANDA membership vote. This includes several activities.

A. The DRC creates a mail ballot of proposed diagnoses to be distributed to all current NANDA members.

B. The DRC oversees the distribution and tallying of ballots. They record any suggestions for needed subsequent revision of any given diagnosis.

C. The DRC communicates information on the outcome of balloting to the original proposer of the diagnoses. Unapproved diagnoses can be revised and can reenter the cycle. Approved diagnoses become a part of the approved NANDA Taxonomy.

D. The DRC forwards the approved diagnoses to the National Conference Proceedings editor for inclusion in the Proceedings and to the Taxonomy Committee for inclusion in the NANDA Taxonomy.

E. The DRC prepares a cycle report for the Board.

Step 8. The cycle is reactivated: The entire diagnosis review cycle is then reactivated. The *NANDA Newsletter* is the official vehicle for communication with the membership about the process, guidelines, timelines, changes, and necessary publicity. Changes in accepted diagnoses undergo this same process and utilize the same review procedures.

*Requirements for Submitting a Proposed New Nursing Diagnosis**

1. *Name:*   A concise phrase, term, or label for the diagnosis.
2. *Definition:*   A clear, precise definition that expresses the essential nature of the diagnosis and delineates its meaning. The definition should enable one to differentiate this diagnosis from all others.
3. *Defining Characteristics:*   A list of observable cues that the client presents when the diagnosis is present. Cues must be both listed and defined, and should be separated into two sets: Major and minor.
   a. Major defining characteristics: Those present in *all* clients experiencing the diagnosis.
   b. Minor defining characteristics: Those present in *many* clients experiencing the diagnosis.
4. *Substantiating/Supportive Materials:*   Minimal validation documentation is a listing of references demonstrating a reasonable review of relevant literature to substantiate the diagnosis. Narrative materials accompanying such a reference list may not exceed 1500 words.

*Adapted from NANDA Development/Submission Guidelines for Proposed New Nursing Diagnoses. There are optional components for submission, and it is suggested that you contact NANDA (address on page 174) for the complete submission guidelines.

Index